MOTHERFOOD

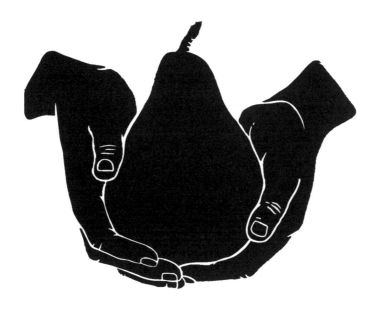

The Science, Art, and Practice
of Nourishing Maternal Foodways

VANESSA A. CLARKSON

This book was written on unceded lands of the Boon Wurrung peoples of the Kulin Nation. We express our gratitude in the sharing of these lands, our sorrow for the personal, spiritual and cultural costs of that sharing and our hope that we may walk together on a just path of healing.

To all mothers, for our mother.

TABLE OF CONTENTS

INTRODUCTION

Thank you. I am deeply honoured that you are here and have chosen to walk with me along this profoundly transformative journey of your life. The path of motherhood will change you in unimaginable ways that you can't possibly foresee.

As you move onto this path, many questions may naturally emerge, including how to nourish yourself well, how to awaken fertility, how to eat safely in pregnancy and how to replenish your body in the newborn weeks and beyond. I hope to explore these with you and, in so doing, unearth the special role that nourishing foods can play in your journey. I also want to take this opportunity to illuminate the many different ways there are of knowing food and, accordingly, light a path that is grounded in respect for your body, compassion, wisdom, humility and, most of all, connection. A path that has been known and walked by our ancestors for the longest time.

To begin expanding our minds I use the term foodways throughout this book. Foodways are our way of relating to food and call us to notice and make sense of our food practices — how is the food grown, produced, exchanged and prepared? How is it eaten and how do our bodies feel about that? And, if there are scraps or leftovers, how are these returned to the Earth to continue the food cycle, or not? Thinking holistically of foodways, rather than reductively of foods or nutrients, nurtures a higher sensibility of our food, our bodies and the Earth.

The humbling realisation that our foodways shape us, just as we shape our foodways, is one of the most revealing gifts from this deepening insight. Humans and nature are fundamentally intertwined and inseparable. And there is no other time in life when this relationship is more apparent than in the peripartum period — during pregnancy and in a baby's first year

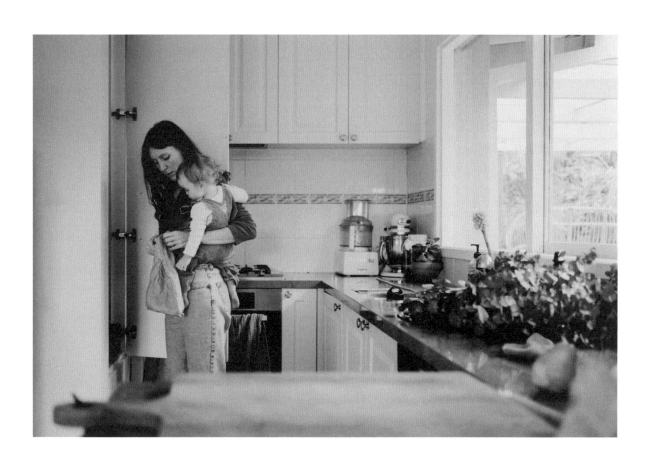

— when the connection between two beings and their foodways is realised and becomes something altogether new — that of a baby and a mother.

It is in the great transitionary seasons of life that we are most open and receptive to exploring new possibilities. Preparing for and having a baby is a time to make sense of our connection with ourselves and the world around us — our interbeing. Yet, motherhood stretches out far before conception and far beyond the birth of a baby. What I share is not bound by linear timeframes nor a label that is granted to us when a baby emerges from our loins. Mother is a verb that we are capable of even if we do not hold a baby in our arms. These are cyclical, universal truths that weave the ultimate connection between people, food and the Earth, that everyone can take notice of. New motherhood simply offers a window through which we can see more clearly the truths that were there all along.

In Chapter 1 — The Science of Motherfood, we journey through the body of knowledge that reveals how the changing nature of connection between people, food and the Earth is what led to the evolution of our species, how we have arrived today in a time of profound disconnection, and how we can start to think about healing this rift. In Chapter 2 — The Art of Motherfood, we look at ways of reimagining lifegiving foodways by thinking about what food practices would look like if they were woven with an approach of care and connection. In Chapter 3 — The Practice of Motherfood, we see a wayfinder — a holistic way of choosing, preparing and enjoying foods so that they nourish us and the Earth. In Chapter 4 — Prepare, we see how our babies embody our foodways, the role of foodways in assuring fertility and begin the groundwork for a nourishing pregnancy. In Chapter 5 — Sense, we notice how pregnancy changes us, learn to take care, to be safe and well in pregnancy, and prepare to welcome a new life. In Chapter 6 — Release, we consider the importance of holding a mother as she explores new ways of tending to her unfamiliar life and go into responsive practices for breastfeeding a newborn. In Chapter 7 — Recipes, we share tried and tested seasonal, plant-based recipes, with further notes on ingredient selection and cooking skills. In Chapter 8 — The Science of

Nutrition, we explore the social life of nutrients, the roles they perform in our bodies, how they work together, and appreciate the interconnectedness between us and the foods we eat. In Chapter 9 — Assist, we look at the place of supplements in times when it is hard to meet nutritional needs through food alone.

I hope this is a book that can be supportive through all seasons of motherhood, contemplative and beyond. Sharing glimpses of ways of relearning and reclaiming the art and practice of nourishing foodways and reconnecting with ourselves by doing so. Mostly, I hope this book assists and empowers you to navigate your own journey, because I believe that we, as a community who mother, have it within ourselves to collectively shape a nourishing future for our children and our mother — Earth.

With our gastronomical growth will come,
inevitably, knowledge and perception of a
hundred other things, but mainly ourselves.

M.F.K FISHER

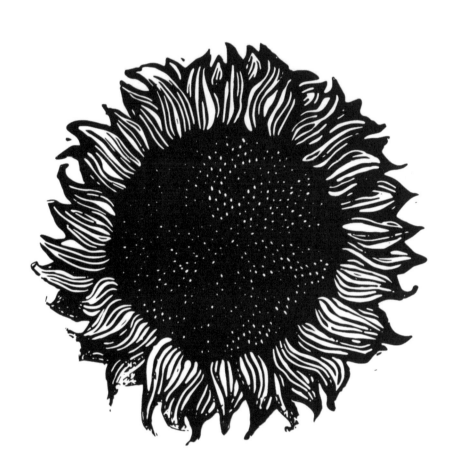

Chapter 1

THE SCIENCE OF MOTHERFOOD

In each and every one of us are the imprints of our ancestral foodways — countless shared meals that have taken place across the ages. We are shaped by these foodways of our deepest past. They are what made us who we are. To understand these deep connections to the web of life is to appreciate our interbeing — our connectedness to all life. This is a science that is rooted in ecology and the study of relationships. A science that reveals that the way we relate to food today profoundly affects life on Earth now and will shape the long-term health of us, our children and the future of all that follow.

Embodying Foodways

On the face of it, the idea that we are shaped by our foodways may not seem profound — the saying 'you are what you eat' is a familiar proverbial lesson. Many people can appreciate that the way we lead our lives, including the foods we eat, impacts our health and well-being. However, what can be more difficult to perceive is that the effects of foodways are not short-lived. They do not start and end with us as individuals. Their force is carried across time from one generation to another, enwrapping us in their wisdom. Our foodways also profoundly shape the world we call home, affecting the lives of many, beyond ourselves.

Becoming Human

When we look at the sprawling diversity of life on Earth today, it is hard to imagine that it all descended from one common ancestor that lived billions of years ago. Humans look considerably different to a worm or an apple, and the wondrous creations of our species — language, art, cuisine, and so on, seem to set us *apart* from nature, but we are *all of each other* — deeply connected through our shared parentage.

Four and a half million years ago, in what is now Africa, our earliest primate relatives would have eaten mostly, if not only, plants. They ate wildly — living in trees and foraging on fruits and leaves, and possibly the odd insect — much like our chimpanzee cousins today. They were physically well suited to their warm, tropical forest homes. They had big back teeth that were good at tearing through hefty amounts of plant material. And their short stature and small brains were readily sustained by the foods available where they lived.

Around two and a half million years ago, the Earth's climate changed to become cooler, drier and more seasonal. In places, these new conditions were unsuitable to sustain the tropical forests of old. The forests shrank and, as a result, our ancestors had to find alternative means of survival, or perish. In place of tropical forests, savanna woodland-grasslands emerged, and these exposed new food options. Our ancestors continued to eat plants, but, whenever possible, animals too.

About two million years ago, the *Homo* group emerged. They retained many of the anatomical features that allowed their tree-dwelling ancestors to digest large amounts of bulky plant foods. However, the *Homo* group were taller, had smaller back teeth, and markedly bigger brains. The only surviving species of the *Homo* group — our own, *Homo sapiens* — have the biggest brains of all; three times larger compared to body size, than our most distant ancestor *Australopithecus*.[1]

Evidence suggests that it was the inclusion of more animal foods — meat and fatty tissue, brain, other organs and bone marrow — that provided the means to support the evolution of nutritionally costly bigger brains. And it was this expanding brain power that enabled our ancestors to develop and exploit new know-how. For example, learning how to make fire, craft tools and cook. Our ancestors became better foragers and in exchange were rewarded with higher nutritional quality in the foods they ate.

We begin to see now that the connection between our ancestors and their foodways is not one-directional but bidirectional. There is a reciprocal relationship to uncover here — an interdependence. This perhaps becomes more apparent when we move onwards in our food story, from prehistory to today.

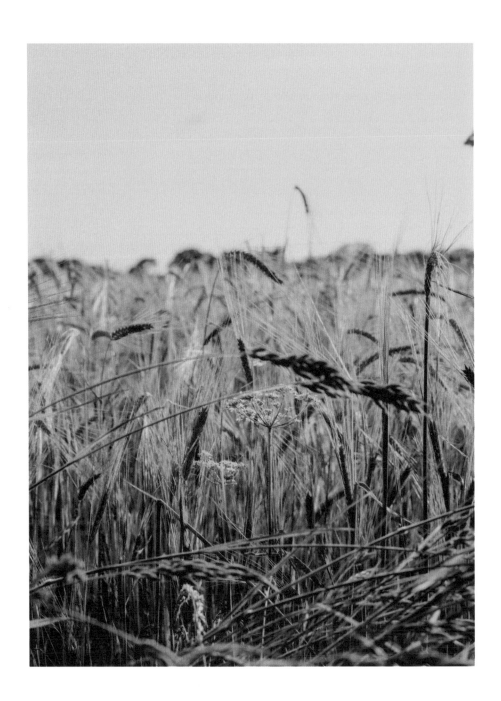

Our *Homo* ancestors continued their nomadic, hunter-gathering way of life for almost 2 million years, but, eventually, new ways of subsisting slowly emerged. From around 12,000 years ago, settlements of agrarian communities began to crop up. First in the Fertile Crescent — a boomerang-shaped region in the Middle East and, independently, later in north and south China, sub-Saharan Africa, south-central Andes, central Mexico and eastern US.[2] Recent research suggests that Indigenous peoples in Australia were practising agriculture prior to colonisation, but when this emerged is unknown.[3] To this day, hunter-gathering remains a way of life for a handful of communities around the world. However for around the last 5000 years, agriculture has been the main way of foodgetting for most of the world's population.

Although it is spoken of as the Agricultural Revolution, the transition to an agrarian way of life did not happen overnight but took thousands of years. The first farmers had to hone the practices involved in cultivating plants and breeding animals for food. With this, the seeds of humankind's dramatic impact on the Earth were sown and the emergence of agriculture marked the first major transformation in the way that humans interacted with the Earth and each other, and both changed as a result.

In general, human health deteriorated with the transition from forager to agrarian lifeways. Agriculture enabled larger groups to settle together and paved the way for early civilisation. However, more mouths to feed meant the food available had to go further and famines were not uncommon. Even then, when food was available, the diversity of what was eaten had significantly diminished compared with forager foodways. Agrarian communities relied heavily on two or three staple grains, including barley, wheat, millet, rice and maize (corn), depending on local ecology. People were generally undernourished, and growth was stunted.

A second major transformation in the relations between humans, and between humans and our ecology, transpired with the industrial revolution in food and farming. Starting around the mid-eighteenth century, the beginnings of a global food trade emerged that centred around wheat.[4]

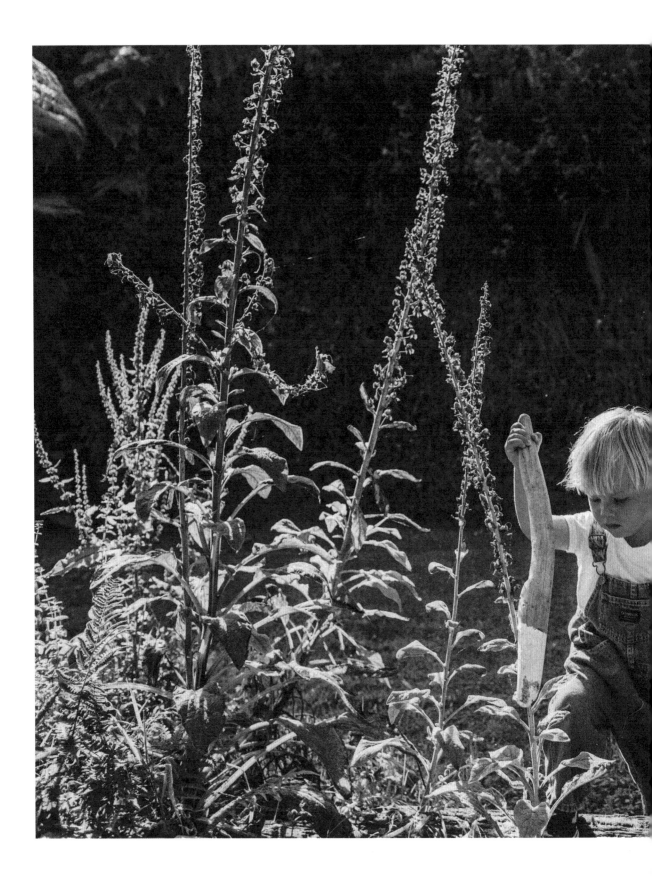

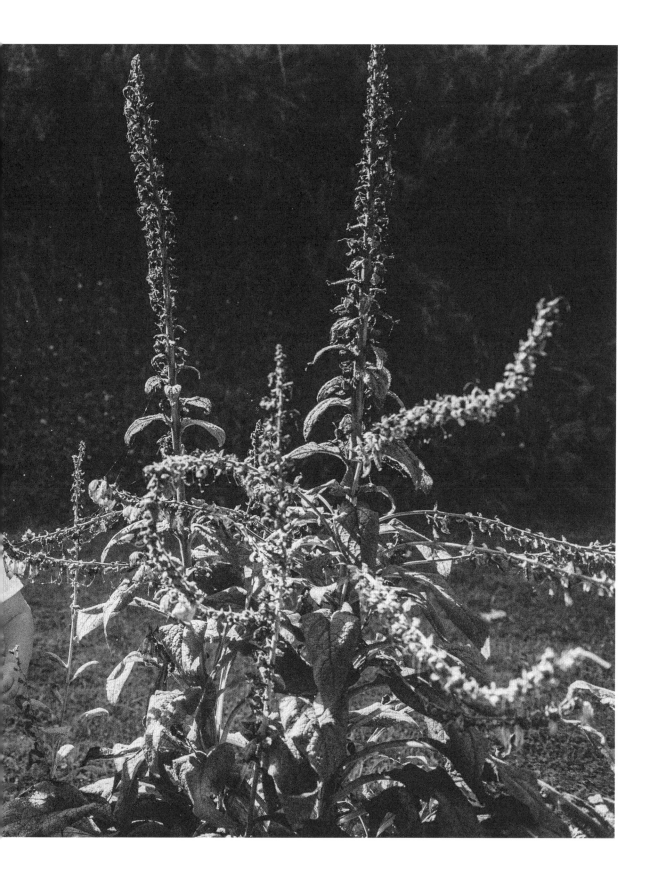

Settler-colonies in North America, Australia, New Zealand and Argentina swept aside peasant farmers — dispossessing Indigenous communities of their land and livelihoods — to make way for the production of cheap wheat and livestock to export to Europe.

After the world wars, the transformation in food and farming accelerated. Food manufacturing capabilities advanced and created an entirely new processed food industry, and a burgeoning mass media industry that convinced people of the wonders of these new 'fast' foods. Broader societal changes both enabled and were enabled by these trends, including the transition of women into the workforce, to work alongside men (rather than in place of them). This meant that ready-made foods found a welcome place in the homes of many who spent more time away from the kitchen than in times gone by.

As we will come to see, the transformation in our foodways over the past three hundred years has significantly affected the health of not just humans, but all life that humans interact with. With each major transition in foodways, the connections between people and between people and the Earth changed, with the overall shift being one of moving further and further away from each other.

In tracing the human origin story and reading of the creative dance between our forebears and their evolving foodways, we can see how entirely intertwined they are. How the foodways of our oldest primate ancestors fundamentally shaped the course of their evolution. And that if they had not eaten what they had, the human species would not exist, and the Earth would not be as it is. It seems that, rather than remarking that 'you are what you eat', it is truer to say that 'you are what your ancestors ate'.

Finding Ourselves

In only 500 generations since the agrarian revolution, we find ourselves now at an evolutionary disjuncture. Our bodies, shaped over the course of two million years of near history, have known nothing but nourishing whole foods for the majority of that time. However, much of the food eaten today looks nothing like the foods to which we are biologically attuned. The modern way of food adversely affects the health of populations, such that billions of people all over the world experience ill-health, and often shortened lives, as a consequence. Our Earth does not fare any better.

Just as the changing climate two and a half million years ago gave rise to new conditions that prompted a shifting of ancestral foodways, we are now at a new precipice. Only this point has not been reached through natural cycles of the Earth's climate, but by human activity. Today, human systems have a degenerative presence on the Earth — extracting as much as possible and in doing so, degrading natural ecosystems, polluting and degrading natural ecosystems and pumping warming greenhouse gases into the atmosphere. These unhealthy human–Earth relations have rapidly and profoundly changed the planet to a point that if things go unaltered, all life faces a bleak future.

Our foodways are the ultimate expression of human–Earth relations. Two-fifths of land on Earth (excluding Antarctica) is used to produce food, and the main way of doing that is causing a significant part of the planet's degradation we are witnessing. Globally, the food system is the largest driver of biodiversity loss and is responsible for 80 per cent of deforestation, more than 70 per cent of freshwater use and produces over 30 per cent of greenhouse gas emissions.[5] The current system of production of animals for food is especially environmentally burdensome; requiring more fossil fuels, land and water than to produce a comparable amount of energy from plant foods.[6] Worldwide, animal production for food provides less than 20 per cent of calories but is responsible for over 50 per cent of greenhouse gas emissions from the food system.[7]

Looking globally, however, hides the unequal burden of upper income countries, who (per person) generally eat far more than their fair share of animal foods and squander significant amounts of the Earth's resources on products that are of little nutritional value, as well as polluting

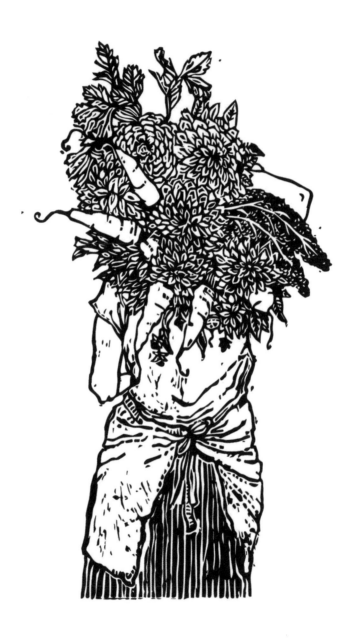

ecosystems with 'forever' plastics and biologically disruptive chemicals. If this wasn't so tragic, it would seem quite a remarkable feat that the food system causes all these issues without even fulfilling its core purpose of nourishing communities.

By now, it is unquestionable that if we are to create a path towards a regenerative human presence on Earth, we will need to change our way of life in relation to food and heal the rift that exists between humans and the Earth. This won't be easy. We cannot go back to the hunter-gatherer ways of our ancestors even if we wanted to — there are too many of us, and not enough wilderness — we'd need somewhere in the order of 15 times the surface area of the planet to eat freely as they did.[8] And our foodways are tangled up in our web of life. We will need to be open to and curious about exploring alternative ways of connecting with food that are currently not familiar to us, or do not, at first, slot seamlessly into our existing lifeways.

Walking On

There is nothing inherently unsustainable about food, just as there is nothing inherently unsustainable about humans. It is just that the industrial system we have constructed to feed ourselves does so in ways that are unsustainable — sometimes through choice, but more often through forces that we don't notice. Our food issues are systemic issues, and that is why our attention should be on cultivating nourishing foodways, not just reductively on food or nutrients. Otherwise, the pace of change will be too slow and fall far short of what is needed for sustainability. These challenges call us to think in a more holistic way.

Just as our ancestors before us, humans can thrive on a wide range of foods. However, there are so many humans now that the choices available to us are narrower than in the past. In times of change, our ancestors put their big brains to good use. They found alternative practices that made them more effective foragers, enabling them to nourish their communities sustainably into the future. We must do that now. We must walk onwards to find foodways that are respectful of the limits of Earth's capacity to nourish us all.

The good news is that there are many possibilities for a food future founded on strong human–Earth relations. With care, the Earth has capacity to nourish everyone without destroying the ecosystems we depend on (and are part of) in the process. Fortunately, motherhood offers a powerful reminder that humans are naturally creative beings.

As we walk on this path of motherhood, our minds naturally open from being focused on nourishing ourselves, to being openly conscious that when we eat, we are nourishing another. Motherhood moves us from a place of egocentrism to ecocentrism — a knowing that humans are equal among all earthly life. That we are not more important and cannot be well-nourished if in doing so, we deplete the very thing from which we draw life. Humans have the capacity to bring forward many possibilities for reorganising ourselves around food, if only we can be aware of and open to them. And, the foodways we seek are not about optimising the health of individuals, but enriching the well-being of all life.

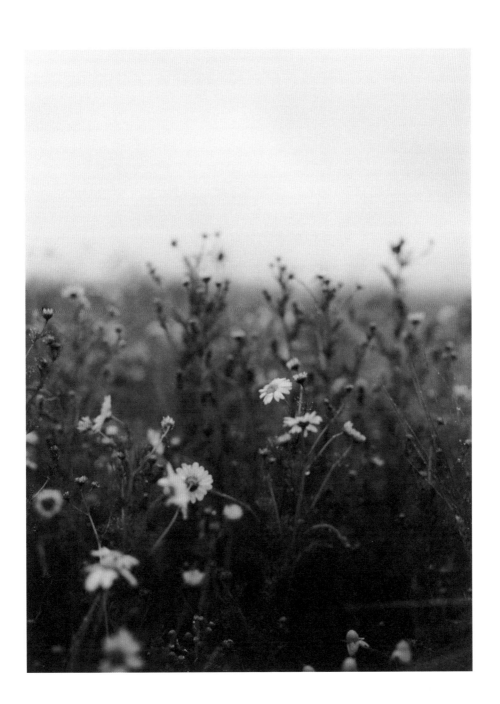

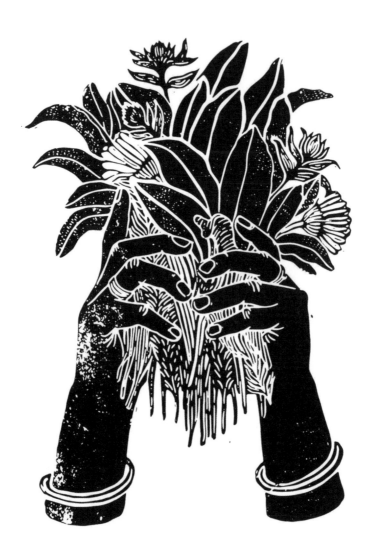

Chapter 2

THE ART OF MOTHERFOOD

When we grow or eat food, we invoke an ancient linkage between ourselves and the Earth, and when we go about exchanging food with others, a kinship is formed that is unmatched by any other social practice. And so, the essence of Motherfood lies in *connection* and the art of Motherfood centres on rebuilding and reaffirming connection to ourselves, each other and the Earth *through* food.

Weaving Foodways

When we are to be guided by connection this calls us to think of weaving — of the many ways there are of tying things together. To *mother* is to weave relationships and as we do so we braid the connections between generations. When mothering, the strands that are chosen guide the strength of the thread and the fabric. Motherfood is woven from two threads: *impermanence* — the wisdom of timeless becoming — that life is forever in constant flux — and *interdependence* — a knowing that humans are inseparable from all other beings. These threads can be tightly woven across all seasons of motherhood, constant and integrative, strengthening and nourishing of each other along the way.

Impermanence

Life is cyclical. Energy rises and falls in a great arc. A perpetual pattern that repeats itself indefinitely and is echoed right across the natural world. Inside the female body, hormones cycle over a month — waxing and preparing her body for ovulation. Then waning and releasing, if conception does not take place. Indeed, the roots of the word *menstruation* come from the Latin word for month and moon. Though not always synchronised, the lunar cycle and menstrual cycle are close to, if not the same length, for many women. Another example is the ample evidence that shows there is a seasonal rhythm in births across human populations, with a rapid increase in conception rate after the spring equinox, that peaks during the summer months.[9, 10]

For our ancestors, the shifting seasons of the Earth and body guided what was eaten. This was a cyclical way of relating to food, listening to and honouring the rhythm of the Earth. To some degree we have lost this art of awareness. Our environment is thick with media and advertising that pushes us to eat a certain way or look a certain way, disinterested in what would nourish the Earth or our bodies. The rhythmical messages from our bodies and nature have been lost to profit-seeking systems that know no value in lifelong nourishment. This distorts our view of and relationship with food and our bodies.

Today, the foods that are eaten often disregard the ecological bounds that we need to live by. Foods are no longer sun-driven. Shops provide the same foods year-round and do this by supplying fruit and vegetables that have been tricked to grow out of season or else by flying them in from faraway places. Where is the break for the chickens who would ordinarily experience an ebb in fertility and egg laying over the winter months? Or for the cows who would not ordinarily produce milk all year? Life is treated like a machine. Yet this is foolhardy. A game ruled by taking rather than co-operating yields benefits only for a few, not for all.

Neglecting the constant flow of life profoundly disconnects us from the Earth, ourselves included. But life is not all summer days. Days flow into nights and summer gives way to autumn. Life is inherently dynamic and cannot sustainably be *take, take, take*. Taking must be balanced by giving. Light evened by dark. This is as true of the Earth, as it is of our bodies. Foodways woven with impermanence are attentive to this wisdom of change. They do not take so much now, so as not to deprive others and future generations from nourishing themselves as well. They are respectful of living within, rather than beyond, the sustaining capacity of their surroundings.

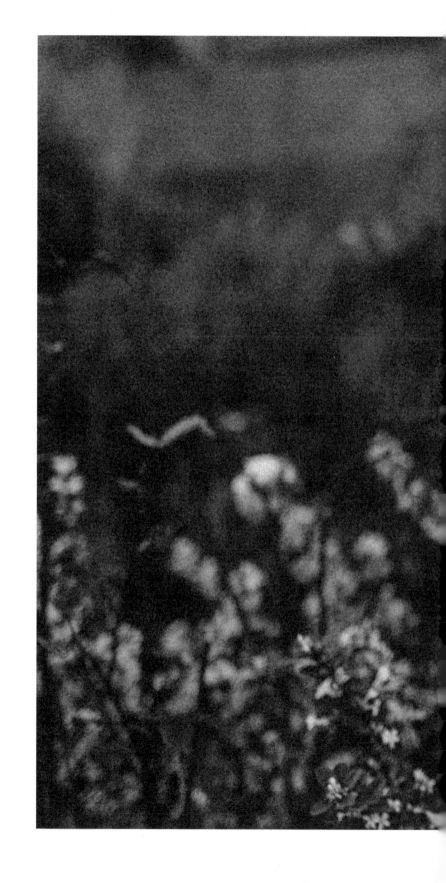

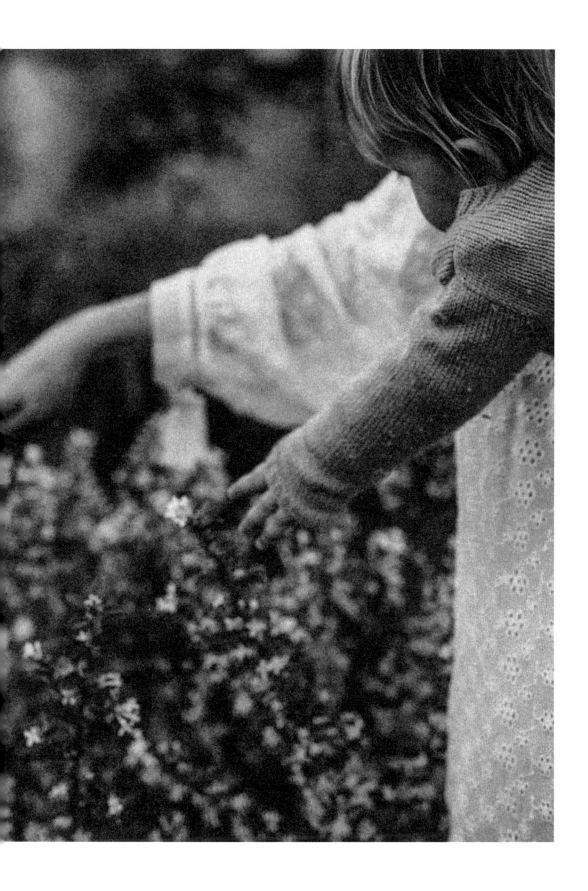

Interdependence

The renowned biologist, Edward O. Wilson once spoke of biodiversity as 'the assembly of life that took a billion years to evolve. It has eaten the storms — folded them into its genes — and created the world that created us. It holds the world steady.' Yet, the world is far from steady now — these are turbulent times. It is estimated that there are 30,000 edible plant species on Earth, yet the food supply is made up of only 150–200 of these.[11] Globally, more than half the energy supplied to humans from food comes from just four staple crops (rice, potatoes, wheat and maize) and only 30 crops account for 95 per cent of food energy consumed.[12, 13]

It wasn't always this way — biodiversity in foodways has declined steeply over the past century or so. An estimated three-quarters of crop varieties vanished between 1900 and 2000.[14] This apocalyptic drop in edible plant species and the simplification of our landscapes is a risky business that has enduring consequences for all life on Earth.

A good example of this is seen when looking inwardly to our guts. It's estimated there are ten times the number of bacteria in our gut than there are cells in our body.[15] But we are not merely hosts to this microscopic community, they are part of us and they play a crucial role in our well-being. Indeed, the Greek root of the word *biome* — the term for this community, translates to *life*. So deeply interconnected are we with our microbiome (little life), that scientists speak of us and our fellow passengers as a *superorganism* — entirely dependent on each other for survival.

Our microbiome performs many vital roles. These include providing immune protection, aiding digestion and making available beneficial compounds that would otherwise be lost to us. When the diversity of our microbiome decreases a little and we lose a few species here and there, this may not matter so much in the grand scheme of life — whatever part they played may be picked up by a similar species that is able to do the same job. But if our microbial community simplifies considerably, the functions of that community can be lost along with it.

Biodiverse foodways cultivate biodiverse microbiomes and conversely, simplified diets from simplified farming systems are echoed by simplified microbiomes. A decline in microbiome biodiversity has now been identified as playing a leading role in the development of many of today's most common ailments, including diabetes, asthma, allergies, coeliac disease, inflammatory bowel diseases, irritable bowel syndrome, bowel cancer, Parkinson's, and Alzheimer's.[16] Communities who have managed to maintain the diversity of their traditional foodways show much lower rates of ill-health connected to the foods they eat.

Foodways woven with interdependence enhance biodiversity. They are respectful of how our foodways nourish us, along with the incalculable communities of beings within and around us. Whether speaking of the immensity of the Earth's one great ecosystem or the minuteness of our gut microbiome, our web of life is utterly dependent on each other for strength, resilience and, ultimately, vitality.

Healing the Rift

As we are guided by these ideas of impermanence and interdependence, we can start to think of ways of restoring connection through food. Our foodways can be reimagined as a circle of practices — producing, exchanging, preparing, eating and disposing — where each practice connects to another, until looping around fully, continuing the cycle. The practices carried out within the *circle of food* are interdependent. For example, the sorts of foods that are grown, and where and how that is done, affects how the food might reach you and what you will do with the food when you have it.

The practices carried out within the circle of food are also interdependent with the world *outside* of these practices, interacting with the lives of other people and the Earth in myriad ways. Weaving nourishing foodways involves thinking holistically about this constellation of food practices and how they are nurturing of healthy relations between ourselves, each other and the Earth, or how they are not. This can take effort, time and, above all, community.

Producing Food

Foodgetting is the most intimate of human–Earth relations.[17] If you can, grow some of your own food — the benefits to mind, body and soul are transformative and immeasurable. When choosing food that others have grown, think about supporting farming systems that cultivate practices that are regenerative and work well with ecology, rather than those that are degenerative and seek to master it.

Regenerative practices enhance biodiversity through mixed farming systems and reforestation, and they conserve water, improve soil health, and use no or very minimal chemical inputs. Regenerative practices are not extractive. They do not take more from the oceans or soils than can be capably replenished. Nor do they deface those ecosystems with plastics and pollutants — for when they do, those plastics and pollutants end up in us and other plants and animals, irreversibly disrupting biology in ways we know so little about. Regenerative practices are respectful of human and animal welfare — they assure the farmhands and fisherfolk that harvest our food have safe and pleasurable working conditions and earn a fair wage, and they afford animals equal care and compassion.

Exchanging Food

With the exchange of food, think of fostering connections between people — bringing together producers and eaters, and supporting farmers in our *foodshed*. Like a watershed, a foodshed encompasses the farming lands and waterways that surround where we live, and which provide a unique ecology from which to cultivate our foodways. Local foods are fresher, more nutritious and usually seasonal, and often don't need shrouding in

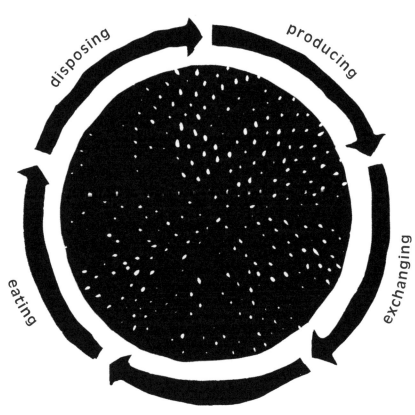

disposing

producing

exchanging

preparing

eating

protective packaging and plastics to make the shorter journey from Earth to plate.

When choosing food from beyond our region, first ask whether it is something that could be grown and produced locally. Doing so can ensure that food is not travelling unnecessarily, adding further to transport-related greenhouse gas emissions. When choosing faraway foods, we can be considerate in our use of them, using only what we need and treating them as a sidekick, rather than the hero on our plates.

Lastly, think about how food is transformed through exchange, including how much processing it has undergone and choosing as close to whole, as often as possible. When reading food labels, begin with the ingredients list — notice from what the product is made and whether these ingredients are familiar to you. You will derive far more connection to food by knowing what is in it and where it was made, than attempting to decipher valueless numbers on a nutrition table. Indeed, in a cultivated pantry, little would bear a label — whole grains, flours and perhaps ground spices at a push.

Preparing Food

Cooking, especially when done with abandon, also teaches us of the personalities of foods in ways that no recipe or label ever shall. Life may get in the way, often more than we would like, but preparing as much food from scratch as time allows, involves us in our foodways, and transforms us in the process. However, food preparation should be practised as a communal affair, otherwise the responsibility has a tendency to rest heavily on the shoulders of women. While there are ways we can lessen the burden of food preparation — batch cooking, using quicker cooking ingredients and so on, it is inevitable that preparing foods from scratch will take up more of the day. The only way to make light and joyful work of cooking is to involve others in the task.

We are fortunate to have available to us a great many culinary ingredients — ready-ground spice blends, pastes, vinegars, oils, wine, pastas, olives and so on, that mean it is not down to us as individuals to nourish ourselves well. There is a raw beauty in that — that a meal before us entwines a community of foodmakers and enriches the lives of many beyond us. When we use these ingredients, we can give thanks to the foodmakers near and far — the humans behind our food. Those who take care to choose quality ingredients and, in doing so, share in our pride and the joy that graces our tables.

Eating Food

Our everyday food practices are largely automatic and paying closer attention to changing our ways of foodgetting is not in our nature. We rely mindlessly on simple cues to determine whether to eat something and to guide how much. Humans, like other animals, have evolved this way because eating is essential for survival and, just like breathing and protective reflexes, practices that are essential for life are more often done instinctively.

Our food spaces — the places where we obtain, prepare and eat our food — are heavily influential in shaping what and how we eat. In the home, we are the custodians of our own food spaces and can cultivate nourishing foodways by tending to our food spaces so they are rich in flavourful whole foods and ingredients, and so they can be enjoyed by others, whenever possible. A strongly woven food culture is grounded in sharing and commensality — sitting with others and conversing over a meal.

Being present and noticing how food makes us feel, matters. We can pause to reflect on the judgements and language we ascribe to foods and question whether these are nurturing of a healthy relationship, or not. Feelings of guilt, shame, restraint and permissibility can all spark tension, driving a wedge in our relationship with our bodies and our food. Negative associations can deaden our enjoyment of both — but motherfood is food for life.

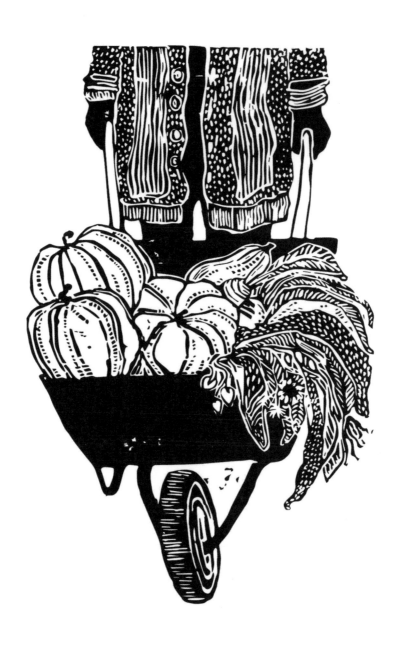

Disposing of Food

We can and should find uses for edible things — chucking food that could have otherwise been eaten squanders all the good that went into producing it to begin with. Added to this is that if food ends up in landfill, it decomposes to produce methane — a highly potent greenhouse gas. Even when attention is paid to using up ingredients before they are past their best and squirrelling leftovers away in diligently labelled containers, there will inevitably be parcels of food left over — woody stalks, bruised leaves and so on. Composting at home or as part of a community-organised or municipal composting scheme reconnects the food circle and cycles the 'waste' back into producing future food.

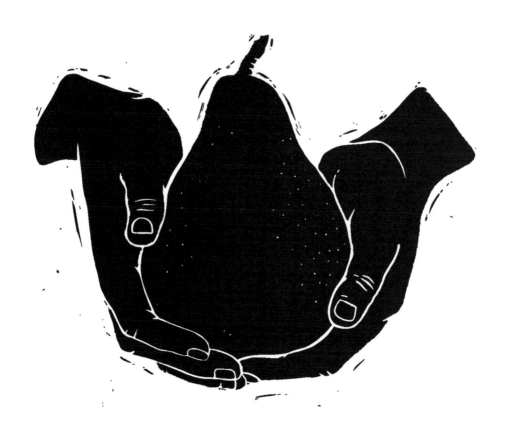

Chapter 3

THE PRACTICE
OF MOTHERFOOD

Nourishment comes in many forms. We can be physically well nourished in a biological sense — when our bodies have all they need. But there is nourishment to be reaped from connection and sharing food with others. From chatting with the farmer who knew the garlic while it grew in the earth for six months. From touching the soil where our food grows, or from feeling the grains as we pour them into the pot. From listening to our bodies and hearing what makes them feel well. From sharing a meal with others. When we (re)connect with food in all these ways, we nourish ourselves fully.

If the art of motherfood is in reconnecting our foodways, then the practice of motherfood is about bringing *connection to life* — exploring ways that we can strengthen our relationship with our bodies, each other and the Earth. What follows is what I know of the practice of Motherfood — thoughts on weaving foodways in the home, that are good and well, and rooted in connection.

Foods from Plants

Plants touch lightly on the Earth and their roots, stems, leaves, fruits and seeds provide the most joyful foundation for nourishing foodways. An abundance of plants can offer so much goodness and provide almost all of what we need to be well. Base your foodways on fresh plants and prioritise those that are locally grown, abundant and seasonal. Fresh fruit and vegetables that have not travelled a great distance to reach you are generally more nutritious, have a lower environmental footprint and support the family farmers in your nearby foodshed. Exploring alternative models of foodgetting may make this a more intuitive practice for you. Examples include veggie boxes, farmers markets, farm gates, community supported agriculture or more traditional greengrocers. Eating this way may not necessarily be more expensive, though if it is, question instead how it is possible to sell food more cheaply. What are the hidden costs of doing so and where have these been offset to?

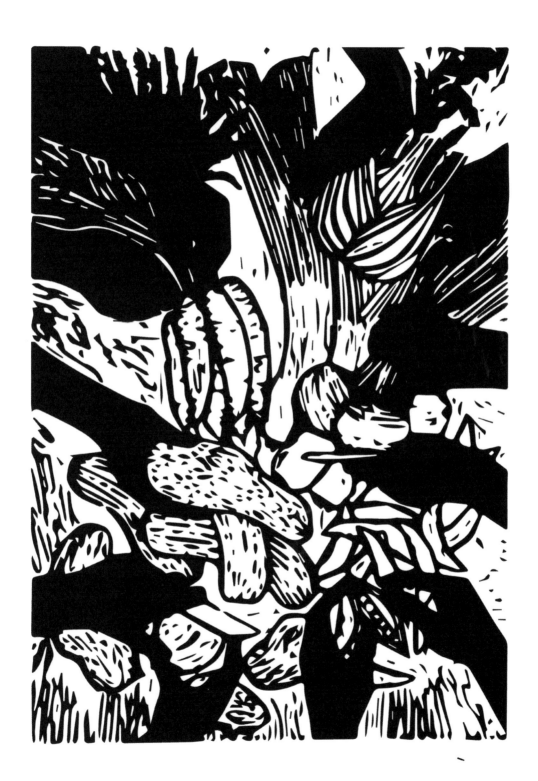

The added benefit of shopping locally/regionally is that with fewer people between you and the farmer, the farmer will inevitably get a larger share of the money you spend. This is important. Farmers are the stewards of the patches of Earth that are dedicated to nourishing our communities. Farmers need to be connected to the communities they serve, valued and financially supported if they are to sustain or transition to ecological farming practices — including fewer or no chemical inputs, such as pesticides.

Pesticides, together with habitat loss or degradation, and climate change are three factors contributing to the alarming decline in insect populations worldwide.[18] In women, pesticides can interfere with reproductive hormonal cycles, and in men, they can negatively affect sperm quality.[19] Pesticides also pass to a baby during pregnancy and breastfeeding, and researchers have raised concerns around the potential for these chemicals to affect a baby's development and long-term health.[20]

Where possible, choose fruit and vegetables that are spray-free and unpackaged. Chosen well, your vegetables may be peppered with soil and tenanted with little critters. But even if they aren't, before you prepare them, always give your produce a really good rinse (and scrub, if needed) under clean, running water.

Leaves and Stems

> Dandelion, nettles, rocket (arugula), mustard greens, spinach, collard greens, silverbeet (chard), mizuna, kale, sorrel, watercress

Starting with the top of the plant, choose the most deeply coloured leaves you can find — greens, reds, purples, and try to eat them at least once a day. In many cases, briefly blanching leafy greens and/or including some lemon juice can take away their bitter edge. Many leafy greens can be grown year-round in temperate climates and, if you can keep the snails away, are easy enough to grow if you have a little space.

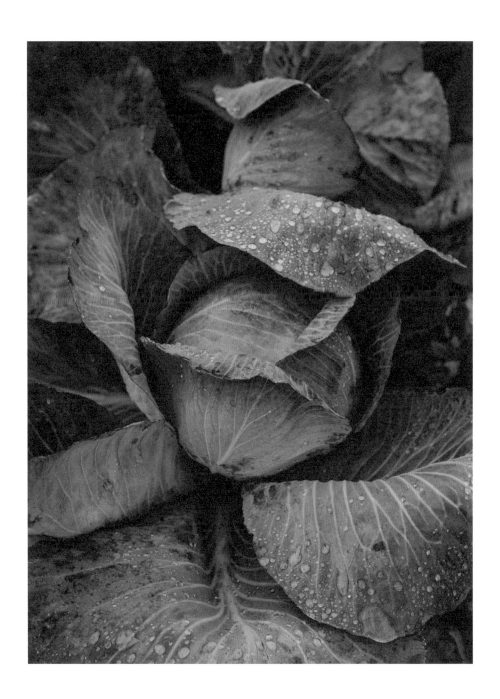

Roots

Beetroot, carrot, celeriac, garlic, ginger, Jerusalem artichoke (sunchokes), kohlrabi, onion, parsnip, potato, radish, sweet potato, turnip

The roots of some vegetables like beetroots, potatoes and parsnips are where they store their energy — making them good in place of grains to round off a hearty meal. Most roots cook well simply roasted in olive oil, honey and a good pinch of salt. They do not need peeling — giving them a good scrub just to shake off the dirt makes sure to keep all their goodness together. Not forgetting, as well, that the leaves of some roots, including carrot and radish tops, turnip and kohlrabi leaves, and beetroot greens, are better sautéed in butter or oil than discarded to the compost heap.

Potatoes are an interesting case, because as a starchy tuber we have a longer history of including this sort of food in our diets than we do grains. However, modern potatoes are very unlike what our ancestors would have eaten. The wild ancestors of modern potatoes, of which there are thousands, originally came from the mountainous region of the Andes. Over the past 8000 years or so, potatoes have been bred to be bigger, milder tasting and incredibly productive as a crop.[21] Unfortunately, through this process their nutrients have also been bred out and now, much of what is left are quickly absorbed carbohydrates that more closely resemble modern, refined grains in terms of the way the body handles them.[22] But, boy, do they taste good.

Fruit

Temperate: apple, pear, berries (e.g. strawberry, raspberry, blackberry, blueberry), stone fruits (e.g. apricot, peach, plum), fig
Subtropical or tropical: banana, guava, mango, pineapple, citrus (e.g. lemon, lime, orange), passionfruit, papaya

When ripe, fruit are good and sweet, and the simplest of foods to eat. Season and ecology will filter the flow of what is available. For example, aside from pome fruit (apples, pears, quince), winter will bring a natural lull. At this time, turn to preserved fruit or other parts of plants, including hardy greens and protected roots — plants that fare well in the cooler months. Summer, in contrast, will be a more abundant time in the home for fruit eating. More often than not, it is best to make the most of fruit and enjoy them whole. When fruit are juiced or blended, they lose a little of themselves, as the tool does a job that your body would benefit from doing.

Sea Vegetables

> *Greens*: sea lettuce
> *Reds*: dulse (dillisk), nori, agar, Irish moss
> *Browns*: kelp, kombu, arame, wakame

Sea vegetables are not quite plants nor animals, but are a form of algae found in all the world's oceans. Nearshore communities have used this marine medicinal since ancient times. Today, sea vegetables, or seaweeds as they are more commonly known, remain holdfast in the traditional foodways of South East Asia and a smattering of other places, including Ireland and Iceland. It is estimated there are over 10,000 kinds of seaweed. Grouped by colour, most of these are red (7000), brown (2000), then green (1000). Seaweeds can be bought fresh (or, if you're lucky, foraged) or dried. When dried, seaweeds can be stored for years in a cool, dark place.

Embodying the mineral-rich water in which they grow, seaweeds are a wonderfully nutritious and flavoursome addition to cooking. With a naturally salty taste, seaweeds can be used in most places I can think of where salt is used as a seasoning. As a general rule, just a little goes a long way. If you're unfamiliar with using seaweeds but are keen to try, a good place to start is using a good pinch of dried dulse in broths, soups or stews.

Seaweeds are particularly high in iodine, a mineral that is crucial to support a baby's growing brain during pregnancy and breastfeeding. Iodine makes seaweeds especially beneficial at this time. Brown seaweeds are especially high in iodine and are best used more sparingly, for example, once a week or so. Seaweeds also absorb pollutants including heavy metals, so ensure you purchase from a reputable supplier — locally, if that is an option for you.

Pulses

> *Beans*: adzuki beans, black beans, borlotti beans, cannellini beans, kidney beans, mung beans, soybeans
> *Lentils*: beluga, French green, lenticchie verdi, Puy
> *Peas*: black-eyed peas, chickpeas (garbanzos) — kabuli and desi

If you have pulses and spices, and a pot of water to cook them in, you will always have a meal — made all the better with onion, vegetables and whole grains but a meal, nonetheless. I keep a range of pulses in my pantry — most of them are dried, but canned or jarred pulses are handy for when time is short. I usually stock up on dried pulses once a quarter through a local bulk buying group and order several kilos of each of my most used. Despite the initial outlay, this way works out more cost-effective over time and minimises packaging.

Preparing pulses according to time-honoured practices makes them easier to digest and cleave nutrients from. Pulses, along with grains, nuts and seeds, contain a compound called phytic acid (also known as phytate). Sometimes referred to as an *anti-nutrient*, phytic acid binds to the minerals found in these foods and prevents them from being absorbed (see also Anti-nutrients, page 285). The more that foodways rely on plants for nutrition, the more attention should be given to reducing phytic acid and maximising mineral absorption.

For the most part, phytic acid is not affected by heat, even at high temperatures (~100°C). Although milling can reduce phytic acid in grains,

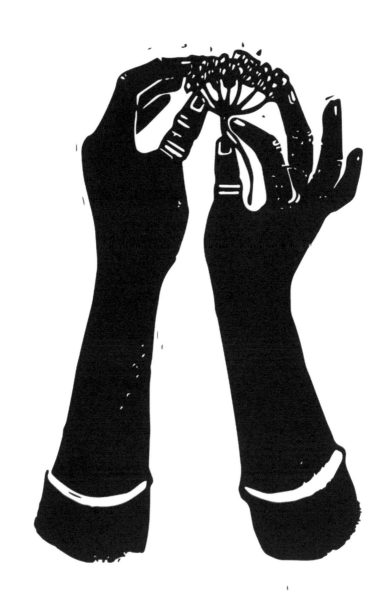

as it is mainly found in the outer layers (note that this is not the case with pulses, where phytic acid is found throughout),[23] this is also where many minerals and fibre are housed — sacrificing nutrients along with the phytic acid is not ideal. Other simple, yet effective, ways of promoting mineral absorption from plant foods like pulses include adding fermented foods and/or fresh fruit and vegetables to meals: fermented foods contain various organic acids that prevent phytic acid binding to minerals and stopping their absorption, while fresh produce is generally high in vitamin C, which can aid iron absorption.[24] Canned pulses usually have lower phytate levels due to their high-temperature cooking and soaking.[25]

Other, more promising, though at times faffy, practices are the three s's — *soaking*, *souring* and *sprouting*. These techniques reduce phytic acid by awakening enzymes that neutralise it.

> *Soaking*: Take a large pot. Pour your pulses or grains into it and cover with lukewarm water. Add a generous pinch of salt to pulses (1 per cent solution, i.e. 10 grams salt per litre water) to help soften them, but not to grains. Instead, grains benefit from souring after soaking (see below) for example, with a little whey, sourdough starter, sauerkraut juice or acid like lemon juice or apple cider vinegar. Set aside in a warm spot for a good amount of time — say 12 hours or so. Overnight, perhaps. As time goes on the phytic acid will leach into the water. Drain, but rescue the water before cooking — it now contains phosphate from the phytic acid, and you can use this mild fertiliser to water your plants, if you like. The pulses and grains are ready to cook, or you can sprout them.

> *Souring*: There are many ways of fermenting-souring pulses, grains and other foods. The essence of the practice lays in transforming foods by various bacteria, fungi and the enzymes they produce.[26] Fermenting can involve cultivating the

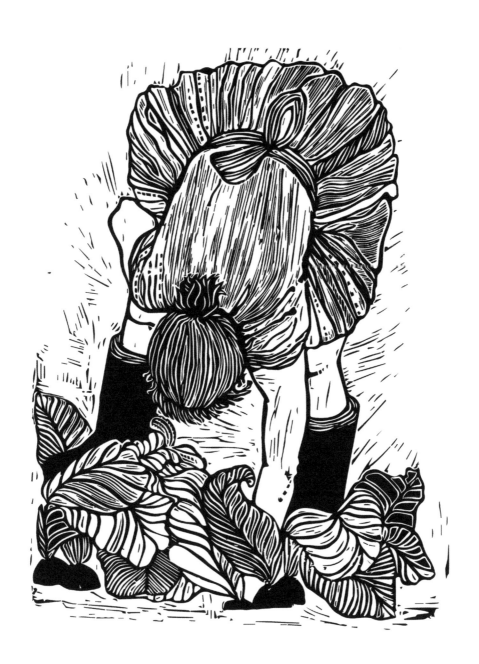

microbiota already living on foods or in the air, known as *wild fermentation*, or purposefully adding a microbial community (also known as a starter) to kickstart the process, known as *culturing*. An example of wild fermentation would be sauerkraut (see Beetroot and Ginger Sauerkraut, page 249) and an example of culturing would be yoghurt or sourdough bread (see Cultured Plant Yoghurts and Cream, page 253).

Sprouting: After soaking, drain and rinse the pulses or grains. Tumble them carefully into a good size jar, with space enough so that some growth is possible. Cover with a breathable cloth, like muslin, and slip a rubber band over the jar's neck to hold the cloth in place. Prop the jar on a slight angle to allow any water to drain out. The next day and the day after, or until shoots appear, rinse and repeat. At this point you can cook the sprouts to your liking or eat them raw. In a salad would be reasonable, maybe with a good squeeze of citrus and toasted nuts or seeds. Or with gently fried spring onions, podded peas and torn mint.

When cooking pulses, a hasty splash of good quality olive oil will create a silky broth and often stop foaming. If the broth is not used straight away, cool and refrigerate for cooking with later. A bay leaf or kombu strip are also good friends to pulses as they cook. Opposite is a general guide to cooking pulses. I watch my pulse pot. If the thirsty pulses poke their heads above the water line, I add a little more water and tuck them back in. Pulses do not need submersing in copious amounts of water when cooking, as all their colour, flavour and nutrients will seep into it.

I usually cook far more pulses than I need and then bundle them into containers and refrigerate or freeze. Lentils take less time than beans (they cook well enough without soaking, though their phytic acid will remain), so I use these more often. Acidic ingredients like tomatoes, vinegar and yoghurt, and salt, can slow down the cooking of pulses and should only be added when tender. As a general rule, dry pulses will yield 2–3 times their original amount when cooked.

Pulse (1 cup)	Water or broth	Stove cook	Pressure cook
Adzuki beans	2–3 cups	1–1½ hours	45 minutes
Black (turtle) beans	2–3 cups	1¼ hours	45 minutes
Cannellini beans	2–3 cups	1–1½ hours	45 minutes
Kidney beans	2–3 cups	1½ hours	1 hour
Mung beans	3–4 cups	1 hour	20 minutes
Split lentils	3 cups	Under 10 minutes	Not recommended
Whole lentils	3–4 cups	20–30 minutes	20 minutes
Chickpeas	3–4 cups	2–3 hours	2–3 hours
Split peas	3–4 cups	1 hour	20 minutes
Whole peas	3–4 cups	3 hours	1 hour

Aquafaba

Aquafaba is the cooking water from chickpeas. It behaves as if it were an egg white — fluffing up and trapping air when you whisk it — though it can be a little more troublesome to set. About 3 tablespoons of aquafaba can fill in for a whole egg, 2 tablespoons for an egg white, and 1 tablespoon for a yolk. I don't always have aquafaba to hand, so you'll find I mostly use flaxseed (linseed) in place of eggs in my recipes.

Grains

> Amaranth, barley, buckwheat, corn (maize), millet, oats, quinoa, rice, rye, sorghum, teff, wheats (e.g. durum, einkorn, emmer [farro], khorasan, spelt)

Grains are seeds of grasses (*Gramineae*). Some of those I have listed (amaranth, buckwheat and quinoa) are not grains in a botanical sense — but their use is similar and so I have included them here. There is huge diversity in the grains that humans have cultivated over millennia. Grains are revered as sacred by many societies — they are filling, nutritious, storable, and grow in almost any climate.

Artefacts suggest grains have been eaten by humans since ancient times. A sandstone pestle studded with oats has been found in a cave in south-eastern Italy.[27] Dated at 33,000 years old, the tool shows old ways of grinding wild grains for flour. Earlier still, 100,000-year-old tools retrieved from a cave in Mozambique were indented with crushed sorghum seeds.[28] However, while these excavations and others pre-date agriculture by tens of thousands of years, collecting and preparing grains was considerably more onerous than foraging for fruit and leaves — especially with primitive tools. Before agrarian lifeways took hold, it is unlikely that grains were a major feature of hunter-gatherer foodways.

Complete grains are made up of three edible layers: an outer layer called the bran (a protective, nutrient-rich sheaf); inwards of this is the germ (a grass seed's equivalent to an egg yolk — home to most of the grain's goodness and from where new life emerges); and at the heart of the grain is the endosperm (a greedy store of mostly starch and some protein that fuels a seedling's growth, before enterprising young roots and leaves are ready to take over).

Whole grain kernels, or those that are coarsely milled or rolled, contain all three layers, making them the most nutritious choice. Further milling and/or sieving yields polished or 'pearled' grains or lighter flours that cook quicker and store for longer. However, they also lose a lot of flavour, and when grains are refined this leaves just the energy store — with no outer layers to slow down the release of energy, refined grains can flood the body with sugar that may be difficult to deal with.

Whole grains have a shorter shelf life than refined grains, as the bran and germ contain oils that go rancid over time. Whole grains will usually keep for up to six months in sealed containers in a cool place, and whole grain flours up to three months. If you have space, whole grain flours and lightly milled grains, such as cracked or bulghur wheat, will keep well in the refrigerator. Refined grains and flours will keep much longer — often up to a year at room temperature.

When cooking, dry toasting a whole grain for a few minutes before adding the water will enhance its nutty flavour. As a rule of thumb, one cup of uncooked whole grains usually yields enough for two people. The table on the following page is a general guide to absorption cooking times and yields for more common grains. If you'd like to add salt when cooking, ¼ teaspoon or less per cup of grain should be ample. If cooking whole grains, add the salt after the grains have softened as it can sometimes toughen the endosperm.

Grain (1 cup)	Water or broth	Stove cook	Pressure cook
Amaranth	1½ cups	25 minutes	5 minutes
Barley — pearl	3 cups	30–60 minutes	35 minutes
Barley — whole	3 cups	1½–2 hours	35 minutes
Buckwheat/kasha	1½–2 cups	10–20 minutes	5 minutes
Bulgur	1½–2 cups	30–40 minutes	10 minutes
Farro — whole	2½ cups	50–60 minutes, soaked 2–3 hours, unsoaked	45 minutes
Millet	2 cups	15 minutes	10–15 minutes
Oat groats	3 cups	1½ hours	30 minutes
Quinoa	2 cups	15–20 minutes	Not recommended
Rice — brown	2–2¼ cups	40–50 minutes	30–40 minutes
Rice — wild	2½–3 cups	50–80 minutes	40–50 minutes
Rice — brown basmati	2 cups	40–50 minutes	40–50 minutes
Rye berries	2½–3 cups	1 hour, soaked 2 hours, unsoaked	40 minutes, soaked 50 minutes, unsoaked
Spelt berries	3 cups	1 hour, soaked 2 hours, unsoaked	40 minutes, soaked 50 minutes, unsoaked
Teff	3–4 cups	15–20 minutes	Not recommended
Wheat berries	2 cups	1½ hours	40 minutes, soaked 50 minutes, unsoaked

Note that rolled oats are generally steamed to prevent rancidity of their oils and enable longer storage times. Look for unstabilised oats (not heat treated) if you plan to soak them to reduce their phytic acid content.

Gluten

> Found in barley, oats,[1] rye, triticale (wheat-rye hybrid), wheats (including spelt)

Certain grains contain a protein called gluten. Most people have no issue with gluten in foods and there is no benefit in avoiding it. However, some people are sensitive to gluten and eating gluten-containing grains is problematic. Coeliac disease is a condition where the body mistakes gluten to be toxic and fires up the immune system to attack it. The resulting inflammation and damage to the gut can cause discomfort and lead to nutritional deficiencies from poor absorption. Coeliac disease is also connected to infertility in both sexes. When the cause of infertility is unknown, it is worthwhile for couples to be screened for this condition.[29] People can also be sensitive to gluten without having coeliac disease.

In theory, managing gluten sensitivities and coeliac disease is straightforward and involves avoiding any foods containing gluten. However, in practice, this can be more of a challenge, particularly as cross-contamination of minute amounts of gluten can still cause damage and discomfort. It is worth pointing out that sometimes symptoms from eating gluten-containing grains may be caused by components other than gluten. In these cases, swapping to gluten-free grains will not help to ease symptoms.

Nuts and Seeds

> *Nuts*: almonds, Brazil nuts, cashews, chestnuts, hazelnuts, pistachios, walnuts
> *Seeds*: chia, flaxseeds (linseeds), hemp, pepitas (pumpkin seeds), sunflower kernels, sesame seeds

---

1   Gluten is the name given to a group of proteins that are digested similarly by people with gluten sensitivity. Oats contain small amounts of avenins — a more easily digested protein of the gluten family. Some people with gluten sensitivity fare okay with oats.

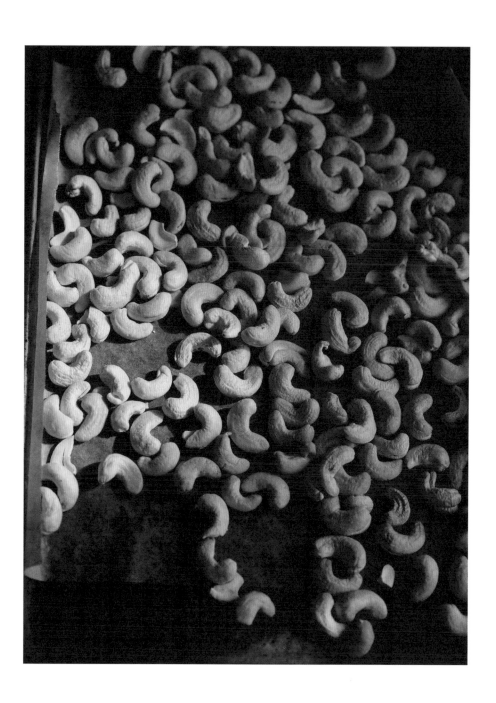

Nuts and seeds can be very different from a flavour and nutritional perspective. It is impossible to talk about them all. At the very least I would encourage you to enjoy as wide a variety as you can manage and a fair handful each day. Nuts and seeds contain sensitive fats that, if left too long, have a tendency to go off. Keep just a small amount and do not replenish them until your supply is all but gone. Buying whole nuts and seeds, and grinding them as and when you need to, is also a good idea. Ground nuts and seeds (like almond meal) quickly go rancid, and it is not uncommon to find ready-ground meals in the shops that have already gone off. You'll need a powerful high-speed food processor to make nuts and seeds into a fine meal or paste.

As a general rule, if you have the space, nuts and seeds are best refrigerated. This has the upside that they are also in plain sight, and I find I reach for them more often. Otherwise, a cool, dark cupboard is good enough. Toasting deepens their flavour, as well as helpfully boosting their nutritional content by making their minerals easier to absorb. Nuts and seeds are best eaten whole. Being rich, they also produce excellent oils.

To make nut or seed butter and milk

To make, first soften the nuts or seeds by soaking them for a good amount of time in water. Overnight will work well. In the morning, drain, rinse and blend into a smooth paste using a food processor — this is your nut or seed butter. For a plant milk, the ratio of nuts or seeds to water is one-part to four-parts, or thereabouts. Less water will give you a creamier result. To make the milk, add water to the smooth paste according to the one-to-four ratio and blend. From here, depending on the power of your blender and the nuts or seeds used, some milks are best strained to clear away any pulpy remnants. This can be done by pouring and squeezing the milk through a clean cloth, like a muslin, or using a mesh strainer and the back of a spoon. Keep the pulp and add this into recipes — there are lots of ideas online. It is worth knowing that cashew and hemp milks are usually good to go without the extra straining step.

Coconut milk

The stem end of coconuts is almost face-like, and it is from this likeness their name originates — the word *coco* is a mythical ghoul in Portuguese and Spanish folklore. The luscious meat of coconuts, when blended with water, produces a sweet milk that is found in most tropical cuisines. It is easy enough to make coconut milk at home by blending fresh coconut or unsweetened, dried coconut (copra) and water. If you gently toast the copra first, the milk will look honeyed and taste as sweet. Good quality coconut milk — that is coconut meat, water, and nothing else — can be bought and kept on hand for use in many dishes including soups and curries. Coconut milk that is gently thickened and cultured, also makes a luscious creamy yoghurt (see page 254).

Tahini

Tahini is a silky, spoonable butter made from raw or toasted sesame seeds. It is widely used in traditional foodways that stretch far and wide across Africa, the Middle East, Asia and India, and finds culinary homes in equally diverse places — from hummus and baba ghanoush, to halva. Sesame butter is the name usually reserved for tahini made from whole (unhulled) sesame seeds, whereas tahini is generally made from hulled seeds, and is usually thinner and milder in flavour. Both are replete in minerals, though unhulled is more so. Tahini is a fine stand-in for nut butter for those with nut allergies (so long as it is processed appropriately to avoid cross-contamination). It will keep longer in the fridge, but this will make it harder and more difficult to drizzle. Recently, health authorities in Australia and New Zealand have advised avoiding tahini during pregnancy due to a small risk of salmonellosis.

Oils

Culinary oils are the juices pressed from fatty nuts and seeds, and fleshy fruits, like coconuts and olives — sometimes called drupes. Just as juicing a fruit discards some of its fibre and nutrients, the same is true when producing oils. Be judicious with their use, favour locally produced and choose as good a quality as your budget will allow.

Oils are made by pressing and can be bottled straight from there or go on for further processing. There are different techniques used to press oils. Some create heat that may damage the sensitive compounds found in the oil. Traditional stone pressing and modern cold pressing avoid this to a reasonable extent and these oils are the highest quality, full of flavour and nutrients, including antioxidants. Hot pressing yields more oil but depletes some of their beneficial compounds. Solvents can also be used to extract oils. In the past, all sorts of questionable chemicals were used, some even carcinogenic. Today, hexane is the main solvent used, though not without concerns over its environmental footprint.[30, 31]

Once an oil is pressed it may be refined further before bottling. Refining removes some colour, flavour and odour, which on first glance doesn't seem like a good idea. However, refining makes oils more stable, enabling them to be stored for longer and used at higher temperatures. Refined oils are also suitable options when you want a more neutral flavour.

After going to some lengths to acquire good quality oils, it is important to use them in ways that maintain their flavour and nutrition. Spoiled oils are rancid and as they decompose will exude an acrid smell. This is what you can smell when you sniff wholemeal flours that have been stored past their best. Oils are entirely fat, so rancidity is especially important to be aware of when choosing, using and storing them. Certain ways of handling oils can hasten their decay. Heating is the big one.

When an oil is burnt it gives off a blueish vapour, releasing toxic compounds including acrolein — the same gas found in tobacco smoke that increases lung cancer risk. Oils will decay at different temperatures known as their smoke point. Oils with a low smoke point, which includes many unrefined oils, should not be used for cooking. Animal fats generally have lower smoke points than vegetable fats, except ghee — butter that has been clarified to remove its milk solids.

Use	Oil	Smoke point
High heat — suitable for all purposes, especially frying and high-temperature baking	Refined oils of avocado, almond, apricot kernel, canola/rapeseed, safflower, corn, palm, peanut, soy, sesame, hazelnut	260–220°C
Medium heat — suitable for sautéing and baking	Refined oils of grapeseed, walnut, coconut	220–180°C
Low–medium heat — suitable for sautéing and baking at a lower temperature	Unrefined oils of peanut, sesame (toasted and untoasted), olive, corn, soy, coconut	180–140°C
No heat	All other unrefined oils, including argan, almond, avocado, flaxseed, hazelnut, pumpkin, safflower, sunflower, walnut	110°C

Adapted from: Wittenberg, M. *The Essential Good Food Guide*, p.222
NB The table is intended as a general guide. The smoke point of oils can decrease with storage and reuse.

Oils will last longer chilled, especially when they are cold pressed and/or unrefined. Choose small bottles made of dark glass. Plastic bottles may contain hormone disrupting chemicals that are more prone to leaching when in contact with fatty/oily foods (see also page 98).[32]

Coconut oil

Coconut oil has earned quite an impressive reputation for being a healthier oil but there is scant evidence to support its marketing claims. Indeed, the studies that have been done point more towards it being less heart-healthy than other plant oils.[33] The use of coconut oil in processed products will not make them healthier. When coconut is eaten in its whole form, as it is in many traditional tropical foodways, it contributes to an overall healthy and sustainable dietary pattern.[34] However, coconut oil, like any other oil, is not a whole food and as such should be used judiciously.

Coconut oil is made by pressing fresh coconut meat to make virgin or extra-virgin coconut oil (terms used interchangeably). The oil can be further refined to remove flavour, odour and 'impurities', making it more stable and suitable for cooking with at higher temperatures. Coconut oil is solid at room temperature and is good for using in places that butter (also a solid fat) would otherwise work. However, I am mindful that the coconut products available to me are not grown locally, but likely come from South East Asia, India, or Central and South America, and this is another reason that I use it sparingly.

Olive oil

Olive trees are remarkably hardy and drought tolerant, and continue to bear olives seasonally for a thousand years. Olive oil has been included in traditional Mediterranean foodways for countless generations, with evidence of cultivation stretching back 6500 years.[35] Virgin olive oil is unrefined and aside from losing some fibre, retains much of the original olive's flavour and nutrition. In order of quality, extra-virgin olive oil is of a slightly higher standard than virgin olive oil, and first pressed olive oil is a luminous green-gold colour. However, the chlorophyll that imparts the green colour is sensitive to light, and it is important to store the oil in a dark bottle/place. Olive oil is produced locally where I live — so it is a choice I will reach for more often than not.

Palm oil

Palm oil is pressed from the plum-size fruit of a variety of palm tree that grows in South East Asia, West Africa, and Central and South America. Palm oil has been used sustainably by traditional cultures for thousands of years — however, the emergence of the industrialised food system has commodified this product and created a global demand for its use in processed food products, cosmetics and as a biofuel. Production of palm oil usually begins with clearing old-growth forests to plant large monoculture palm plantations. In Indonesia, Malaysia and Papua New Guinea, where most globally traded

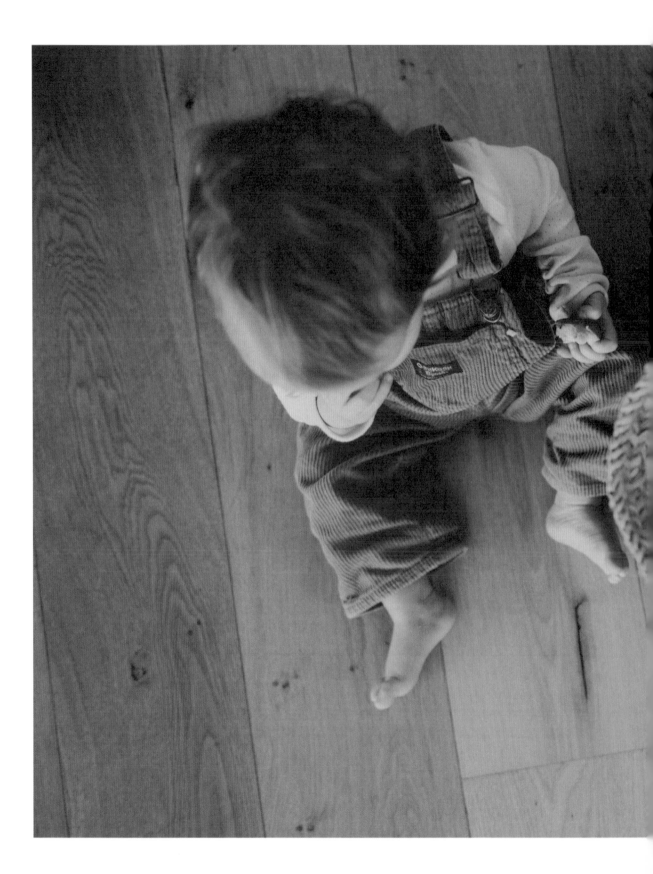

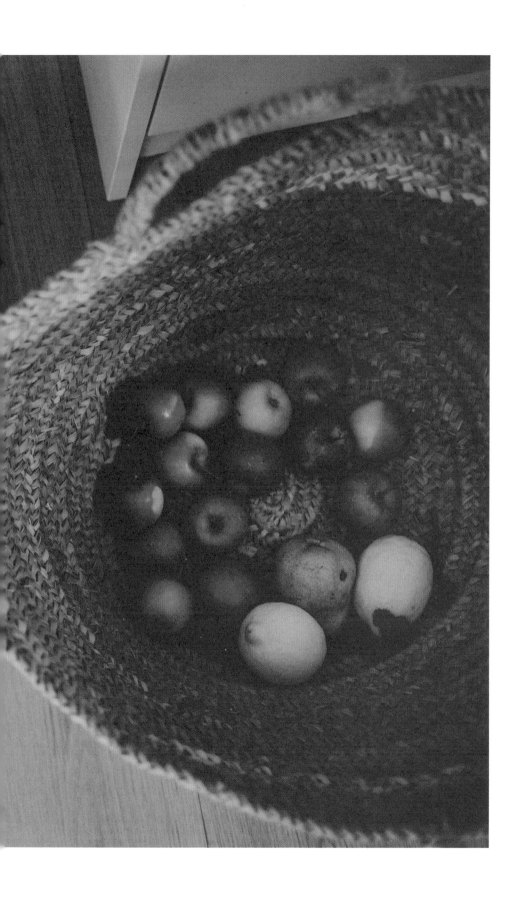

palm oil comes from, such deforestation has endangered the three remaining species of orangutan. There are many other social and environmental issues connected with palm oil production, including human rights violations, land and water pollution, and greenhouse gas emissions (though these are not unique to palm oil and are more a general feature of this way of producing food). While it is possible to find products that are made with palm oil that is 'certified' as being sustainable, independent research shows that such industry-led schemes have not halted deforestation.[36, 37]

Sweeteners

> Honey, maple syrup, molasses, rapadura/panela/piloncillo, palm sugar

All humans have a sweet tooth — it is something we are born with (and never leaves us) and ensures we take well to our first food — our mother's milk. Granted, some may like sweet foods less than others, but the *liking* of sweetness is universal. The modern food system is awash with sweeteners of all kinds, though refined white sugar from cane or beet is most common. And while sugar is used as a cheap way of enhancing the flavour of all manner of foods, the main sources of it would probably not surprise most people — sugary drinks, cakes, biscuits and confectionery.

The sugars found within whole foods like fruit are, reductively and nutritionally speaking, no different from the sugars found in the bags of sugar that line supermarket shelves. However, humans do not fare well with liberal amounts of *added* sugars, as this is not what our bodies are used to in an evolutionary sense. Added sugars add extra energy with little to no nutrition and sugar 'delivered' to the body in this simplified way more often quickly floods the bloodstream and puts pressure on the body to release insulin to clear it. This burden is particularly problematic if there is an intolerance to carbohydrates, as there is with several types of diabetes.[38]

Whenever possible, enjoy using seasonally fresh or dried fruit to sweeten and add flavour to dishes. However, some recipes can't be made without sweetness in its simpler form and granulated sugar, of the kind our grandmas would have used, is imperative for a healthy jam economy — for making homemade preserves, cakes, chutneys, biscuits and so on. This to me, is an altogether different matter and something to applaud as part of connected foodways.

There are now well over a hundred sweeteners available — too many to go through individually. However, I will talk to a few that I like to keep on hand and use more often. I am talking here of sweeteners that come from nature and provide energy, rather than those made in a lab that do not, such as calorie-free synthetic sweeteners. Like all ingredients, the sweetener I choose depends on what I have planned for it, and I use just enough, but no more.

Sugar from cane or beet

There are unrefined versions of sugar available — these artisan products go by many names including *rapadura*, *panela* or *dulce* in Latin America, *piloncillo* in Mexico, *jaggery* or *gur* in India, and *muscovado* elsewhere. They are mostly made from sugar cane, though date palm sap is another option. Despite their many different names, the way these sugars are made is quite similar and is a simple process that doesn't take long to explain. Firstly, the sugar cane is pressed to release its juice. Then it is heated just enough to boil it down to a thick syrup, and from there it is poured into a mould to harden, or it is cooled and beaten into granules.

Rapadura contains more nutrients than refined white sugar (though still only relatively small amounts) but more importantly, it has a rich, caramel flavour that really adds to the dishes made with it. Although brown and raw sugar look somewhat similar to rapadura, they are not the same. These products usually undergo the same extensive processing that is used to produce refined, white sugar but have had some of the molasses added back in for colour and flavour.

Sugar cane is grown in tropical regions and beet, temperate. If your cane sugar has come from a lower- or middle-income country, look for an independent certification mark like Bonsucro, that points to some semblance of fair work and environmental stewardship practices. However, be aware that in the main, producing sugar through conventional industrial scale practices uses a lot of water and fossil fuel-derived agrochemicals, like fertilisers and pesticides.

Honey

If 'modern' hunter-gatherers are anything to go by, our ancestors would have very likely gone to great lengths to acquire wild honey, and the art of beekeeping may have been practised since at least the time of Ancient Egypt. It takes 12 worker bees their whole life to make one teaspoon of honey and for that reason I am not frivolous with it. Raw local honey is the main syrup I use in cooking — if there was ever to be a 'taste of place', it is sure to be found in a small pot of local honey.[2] The floral notes of banksia and yellow box, and arboreal flavours of eucalypt, are happily spooned into my baking, while simpler flavours make it into other meals. Raw honey is not processed and contains probiotic bacteria and small amounts of nutrients and enzymes. Babies under one should not have honey because of a very slight chance of botulism, but you needn't avoid it if you are pregnant or breastfeeding. I am unaware of any evidence to suggest there is a risk to women who eat raw honey during pregnancy.

Maple syrup

There are just a handful of trees that produce a watery sap that can be tapped and boiled down to a thick syrup. Maple is one. Birch another, though less commonly available. The tropics have the various palm tree species and other warmer climes have agave. The practice of making maple

---

2   Although honey is made by bees, I have included it in this section on sweeteners from plants for simplicity. In any case, as honey is the essence of flowers and tree blossoms, its inclusion does not seem out of place.

syrup was, and remains, engrained in the traditional foodways and culture of Indigenous peoples in North America, where they celebrate the 'first tap' and arrival of springtime through song and ceremony. The maple season is short — no longer than six weeks. And from where I live in Australia, maple syrup must travel well over ten thousand miles to reach me. I use it less now than in the past; respectful of that journey and the environmental footprint it confers.

Maple syrup is graded by colour, with the darker shades prized for their complex caramel flavour. Practically speaking, maple syrup can be used in all the same places as honey and even churned into sweet butter in a similar fashion to creamed honey. As well, the sugars in maple syrup are absorbed relatively slowly and invoke a calmer response by the body when they are absorbed (in contrast to most refined sugars).[39] Look out for charlatan 'maple-like' products. As you might suspect, these are inferior to the real deal and are best avoided.

Dates

Fresh and soft (khalal): Medjool, Bahree, Khalas
Ripe and semi-soft (rutub): Deglet Noor, Zahidi
Cured and dry (tamar): Thoory

When not needing a spoonful of sugar or drizzle of syrup, dates can work well in many other places where a caramelly sweetness is called for. Chopped up into tagines and grainy salads or pitted and stuffed with nut or seed butters or all manner of cheeses — the versatility of dates makes them a valuable addition to any kitchen. There are thousands of cultivars of date, but the large and tender Medjools are the most common fresh variety you will likely come across, as well as many nondescript dried varieties that can be stored in the pantry. Dates can also be bought pre-ground into a coarse powder known as date sugar. Note that the Chinese red date (jujube) is botanically unrelated.

Seasonings

To me, a well-stocked pantry is not one where we are tripping over bags spilling with grains or pulses, or where we have more spices than the Silk Roads. Rather, it is a storeroom or cupboard that is considered — where we have good amounts of the seasonings that we use mostly and a little of those that we use from time to time.

The world of fresh and dry herbs and spices, salts, vinegars and other condiments is worth getting lost in. I cannot do the flavourful landscape justice here, but I will briefly cover or list those items that I think are worth keeping on hand.

Miso

Miso is a thick paste made from cooked soybeans or chickpeas mixed with water, salt and koji. Koji is a mixture of grains, usually rice or barley, or cooked soybeans that have been inoculated with *Aspergillus oryzae*, a mould which starts the fermentation process. Miso can be used in marinades, dressings, sauces, spreads, porridge and, of course, soup. Unpasteurised miso contains beneficial bacteria and to keep these intact, avoid cooking with it at high temperatures for long periods — adding miso at the end of cooking will make the most of its flavour. In a similar vein, miso should be refrigerated and will keep for years this way.

There are different types of miso that vary according to how long they have been aged for and their recipes. However, they can broadly be grouped into light and dark:

Light miso: With a shorter fermentation time (one year or less) and less salt, light miso has a sweeter and more mellow flavour than dark miso. Examples include white (shiro), yellow (shinsu) and chickpea miso.

Dark miso: Longer fermentation times (upwards of one year to three years) yield a miso with deeper, more complex flavours than light miso. Examples include mugi (barley), hatcho (soybeans), soba (buckwheat), aka (red rice), kome (white rice), genmai (brown rice) miso. Try my Miso, Ginger and Barley Broth recipe with mugi miso on page 205.

Salt

Salt is the essence of our oceans — where the water has been evaporated and impurities removed. Unrefined, it embodies the minerals from the area in which it is harvested. Sea salt comes from oceans, and ultimately the rocks that erode into them, and rock salt from inland salt mines, where the deposits are remnants of ancient salt lakes and oceans. Long before canning and refrigeration was invented, salt allowed traditional cultures to preserve foods which saw them through seasonal lulls in provisions. But more than that, salt enhances flavour in ways unmatched by any other ingredient.

Salt can be prepared in different ways to produce fine, even crystals (granulated table salt) or larger, flat, irregular flakes, or gravelly chunks. The former works well in baking, when you want an even dispersal of the ingredient through batters and dough. Whereas chunkier salt can be used in general cooking or as a garnish. Salt that is tinted pink, black or grey contains a small amount of trace minerals, which impart this colour and affect the flavour. Iodised salt is available for those who may not ordinarily get enough iodine from their foodways for various reasons (see also Micronutrients/Iodine, page 296).

I could stand for a long time in front of the multiple shelves of salt in our nearby speciality food store — there is a huge array on offer. In the main though, I opt for as local as possible and a mix of fine and flaky that I flip between depending on what is happening in my kitchen.

Salt is made of sodium and chloride, and it is the sodium part that is essential for nerve transmission and maintaining fluid balance and blood pressure. Humans have evolved to expect very little sodium from their foodways, consequently very little sodium is needed for these purposes — around 500–1000 mg (0.5–1 g) per day for adults, which equates to 1.3–2.5 g of salt. Today, most of the salt that is eaten comes from processed and fast foods.

Spice blends

I keep a mix of dried herbs and spices in my pantry — mostly spices, as I grow several herbs fresh. Some of my favourites include cumin (ground and seeds), coriander (ground and seeds), bay leaves, oregano, thyme, turmeric, chilli (a mix of intensities, ground), paprika (smoked and sweet), cinnamon, vanilla (ground and pods), cardamom (ground and pods), ginger, star anise, peppercorns and mustard seeds. Spice blends are a good choice to keep, both economically and for flair, as a skilled foodmaker has taken time to mix complementary flavours together on your behalf. Opposite is a list of some commonly found spice blends.

Other seasonings

SAUCES

Soy sauces — tamari and shoyu
Worcestershire sauce

VINEGARS

Wine vinegars, e.g. balsamic vinegar
Cider vinegars, e.g. apple cider vinegar
Fruit vinegars, e.g. raspberry vinegar
Grain vinegars, e.g. malt vinegar, rice vinegar

MISCELLANEOUS

Baking powder, aluminium free
Bicarbonate of soda
Nutritional yeast (grown with B12)
Mirin

France	
Bouquet garni	Bay, thyme, parsley
Fines herbes	Tarragon, chervil, chive
Quatre épices	Black pepper, nutmeg, clove, ginger or cinnamon
Herbes de Provence	Thyme, marjoram, fennel, basil, rosemary, lavender
North Africa	
Berbere	Coriander, shallots, paprika, black pepper, japones pepper, garlic, fenugreek, ginger, turmeric, allspice, nutmeg, cardamom, cumin, cinnamon, cloves, thyme
Chermoula	Onion, garlic, coriander leaf, chilli, cumin, black pepper, saffron
Ras el hanout	Often includes cardamom, cassia, mace, clove, cumin, chilli, rose petals, and many more
Middle East	
Baharat	Cumin, allspice, black pepper, coriander, nutmeg, cinnamon, paprika, clove, cardamom
Za'atar	Marjoram, oregano, thyme, sesame, sumac
Zhug	Cumin, cardamom, garlic, chilli
India	
Garam masala	Cumin, coriander, cardamom, black pepper, clove, mace, cinnamon
Panch phoran	Cumin, fennel, nigella, fenugreek, mustard
China	
Five-spice	Star anise, Sichuan pepper, cassia, clove, fennel
Japan	
Togarashi	Korean chilli, orange, poppyseed, black and white sesame, paprika, seaweed, ginger
Mexico	
Recado rojo	Annatto, Mexican oregano, cumin, clove, cinnamon, black pepper, allspice, garlic, salt

Drinks

Sweetened Drinks

As a general rule, it is best to avoid sweetened drinks. Those that are sweetened with sugar, whether from sugar beet or cane, or other 'natural' sources like coconut nectar, rapidly flood the bloodstream with large amounts of sugar, which the body is ill-equipped to deal with (see also Bringing Balance, page 95). And while there are many sugar-free alternative drinks that are sweetened with synthetic sweeteners, which contain fewer of the 'empty calories' of sugar sweetened drinks, it is questionable whether they offer a genuinely healthier choice and support weight management in the way that they are intended to.[40] Emerging evidence also points to some synthetic sweeteners (including saccharin, sucralose and several polyols) affecting the gut microbiome.[41] Lastly, synthetic sweeteners have been found in treated wastewater, raising concerns that once excreted from the body they pollute aquatic ecosystems.[42]

Caffeinated Drinks

Caffeine is found in over 60 plant species, including coffee beans, cacao beans, tea leaves, guarana berries, kola nuts and yerba mate. It is possible that caffeine and caffeine-like compounds are made by some plants as protection against insects — a natural pesticide if you like. Caffeine is similarly toxic to humans, but only in very high doses. In small doses, caffeine has a stimulatory effect — promoting wakefulness, lifting concentration, and increasing short-term blood pressure. While people have enjoyed foods and drinks containing caffeine for thousands of years, it's advisable to be mindful of the amounts generally consumed, especially in the pre- and peripartum periods.

Pre-conception

Moderate caffeine intakes do not seem to reduce the chance of becoming pregnant. However, in women, caffeine can interfere with oestrogen levels, as the compounds share the same metabolic pathway and high caffeine intakes have been linked to shorter menstrual cycles.[43] In men, some studies have found that higher caffeine intakes can delay the time it takes to conceive.[44] On balance, caffeine seems okay to have in moderation in the pre-conception period, but as a couple, if you are having difficulty in conceiving, then it is sensible for you both to avoid it.

Pregnancy

In the womb, babies do not have the necessary enzymes to metabolise caffeine, and during pregnancy, the clearance of caffeine from a mother's blood slows down — meaning that a baby can be exposed to caffeine for long periods of time. Moderate caffeine intakes in pregnant women do not appear to affect the long-term health of their babies. However, public health organisations recommend that caffeine intakes should be below 200–300 mg a day (2–3 cups of coffee) pre-conceptually and during pregnancy.[45, 46]

Breastfeeding

The advice for consuming caffeine when breastfeeding is the same as for pre-conception and during pregnancy. Caffeine passes into breast milk, peaking between 1 and 2 hours after ingestion. Some babies can be sensitive to a mother's caffeine intake even at moderate levels, causing them to become restless or kept awake — although the evidence is limited.[47] If you would like to reduce your caffeine intake, be careful to do so gradually. The side effects of sudden caffeine withdrawal can be unpleasant and include piercing headaches, drowsiness, irritability and difficulty concentrating. Keep in mind as well that although tea contains less caffeine than coffee, it still contains tannins — substances which block the absorption of iron and other minerals. Tea and coffee can halve the amount of iron absorbed from foods. If you eat little or no fleshy animal foods, especially dark meat, it is a good idea to minimise tea and coffee consumption to enhance iron absorption (see also Anti-nutrients, page 285). Space out any caffeine drinks between meals to maximise the absorption of nutrients from your food.

Caffeine sources

Black tea (250-ml mug) — 50 mg
Green tea (250-ml mug) — 35 mg
Coffee (1 shot espresso or 1 x 250-ml mug filter) — 140 mg
Hot chocolate (250-ml mug) — 10 mg
Kombucha (200-ml glass) — 10 mg
Dark chocolate bar (50-g bar) — 25 mg
Cola drink (375-ml can) — 50 mg
NB These figures are provided as a guide. Actual levels may vary.

Alcoholic Drinks

Drinking alcohol has both immediate and long-term health effects, with the risk of harm increasing with more alcohol consumed and increased frequency. Heavy drinking (either routine drinking or occasional binge drinking) is strongly discouraged at any time of life but especially so in the pre- and peripartum period. General recommendations for adults are that alcohol should be no more than 10 standard drinks per week and no more than 4 standard drinks in a day.

Standard alcoholic drinks

Light beer (2.7% alc/vol) — 425 ml
Mid-strength beer (3.5% alc/vol) — 375 ml
Full-strength beer (4.9% alc/vol) — 285 ml
Regular cider (4.9% alc/vol) — 285 ml
Wine (13% alc/vol) — 100 ml
Fortified wine (20% alc/vol) — 60 ml
Spirits (40% alc/vol) — 30 ml

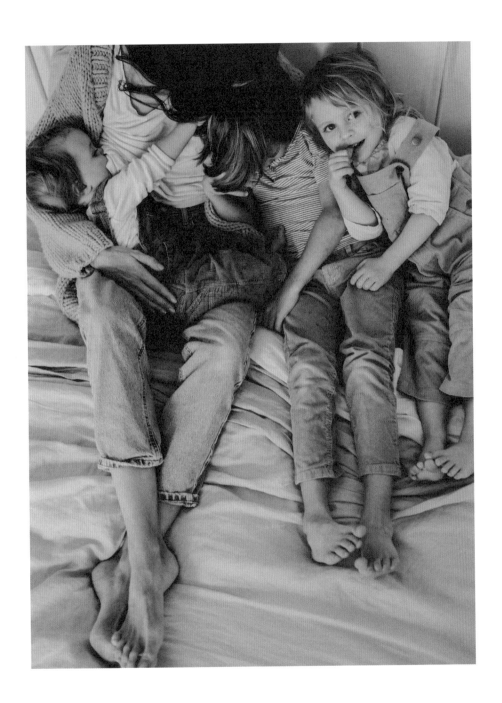

Pre-conception

High alcohol intakes can affect fertility by significantly disrupting the menstrual cycle and diminishing the store of eggs.[48] In men, alcohol disturbs hormonal rhythms, particularly testosterone, and also decreases sperm quality.[49] In contrast to heavy drinking, the effects of low to moderate levels of alcohol consumption (roughly one standard drink per day for women, two drinks per day for men) are unclear and that is why there are conflicting recommendations about what is best pre-conceptually. Similar to caffeine, alcohol in moderation in the pre-conception period probably presents a low risk of ill health effects, but as a couple, if you are having difficulty conceiving, then it is sensible for you both to avoid it.

Pregnancy

In pregnancy, alcohol freely crosses the placenta, and it also accumulates in the amniotic fluid. Babies cannot metabolise alcohol as effectively as adults, and because alcohol is teratogenic, drinking it causes health risks. Heavy drinking in pregnancy can lead to foetal alcohol syndrome. But even moderate intakes of more than 2–4 drinks a week have been shown in some studies to increase the risk of miscarriage, particularly in early pregnancy. As there is no consensus on a safe level of drinking alcohol during pregnancy, it is best to avoid drinking any at all.

Breastfeeding

It is safest not to drink alcohol when breastfeeding. However, if you do decide to drink alcohol, wait until breastfeeding is established (usually after a month) and limit the amount you have — no more than two standard drinks a day. Alcohol passes into breast milk, with the highest level occurring between 30 and 90 minutes after drinking, so it is wise to space drinking away from usual feeding times. It is also worth noting that even though it is customary in some cultures to give beer to breastfeeding mothers to promote milk supply, evidence suggests that alcohol may actually reduce breast milk production.

Foods from Animals

When humans eat animals, they are also eating the animals and the plants the animals ate — they are taking more from the Earth than if the humans were to eat the plants directly. This is one of the reasons why eating diets comprised mostly of plants generally has a lower environmental footprint. Yet we should be careful to distinguish between plants and animals so simplistically. Though, on the face of things, animals seem to take more, they also give back by transforming, concentrating and recycling nutrients, which can then enrich the soil and sustain new plant growth — continuing the food circle. This is the way of the harmonious interaction between plants and animals that is as old as time. Many home gardeners can attest that it is harder (without the help of synthetic fertilisers) to grow foods aptly without replenishing the soil with some sort of animal product such as blood, bonemeal or excrement. The same can be said of humans — when animal foods are eaten, humans benefit from the prework of animals to assimilate and concentrate nutrients in their bodies, milk and eggs. Though it is not impossible to meet nutritional needs without eating animal foods, their inclusion, even in just small amounts, makes it easier to do so.

If animal foods are the way for you, their inclusion should be wrought with care and compassion for the animals — consideration for how well nourished the animals are — physically and mentally. Free range, organic and preferably regenerative animal farming practices connect the animals with natural environments and support instinctive behaviours in ways that intensive systems cannot come close to.[3] Knowing your producer, buying locally and/or researching the practices of the farms that produce your meat, milk and eggs will provide reassurance that your money is not going towards systems that compromise compassion for convenience.

---

3   Grass-fed extensive farming systems can fix carbon into the soil (sequestration) and lead to several other benefits, but these have to be weighed against alternative uses for the land, including reforestation.

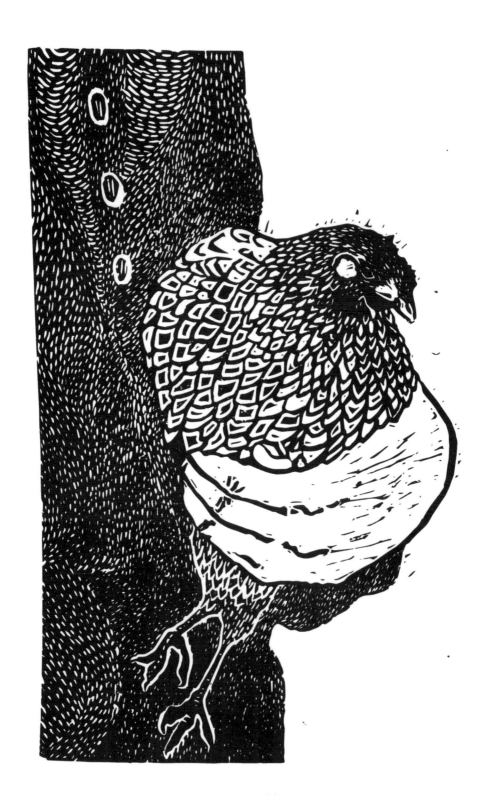

A lot of time, effort and resource, not to mention a life, goes into producing animal foods and this should be reflected in their judicious use. Using as much that is edible as possible, including saving bones to make broth and seeking out undervalued cuts and organ meats, returns true value to the cost of animal foods. Favouring unprocessed or minimally processed meat and dairy products is also recommended. We have a relatively short history of making and eating processed meats. The World Health Organization classifies processed meat as carcinogenic, as research shows that eating it is linked to an increased risk of cancer in the gut (colorectal). Processed meats include bacon, ham, sausages and hot dogs, and differ from unprocessed meats, in containing various compounds that are formed through salting, curing, fermenting, smoking and high-temperature cooking.

Fish and Seafood

Fish and seafood are natural, wholesome and have long been part of ancestral foodways. Today, many coastal communities continue to enjoy large amounts of fish, and fisheries are an essential part of their local economies. Nutritionally, fish are rich in beneficial compounds including very long chain omega-3 fats, vitamin D, iodine and many more.

On the other hand, fish also contain environmental pollutants at levels much higher than our ancestors would have likely been exposed to. One example is methylmercury, a heavy metal which has always naturally been present in small amounts in the environment — as human activities such as mining, coal burning and manufacturing have increased, it has accumulated over time. Also to consider is that since the 1950s, the number of collapsed fish stocks has increased exponentially due to decades of overfishing and destructive fishing practices, and there are over 100 cases of marine population extinctions worldwide.[50] Farming fish is not a solution to declining wild stocks — most farmed fish are carnivorous, requiring more fish feed inputs (fish meal and fish oil) than is harvested.[51]

Polluting aquaculture practices and higher levels of contaminants can also be a problem with some operators.[52]

When choosing wild-caught fish, look for the Marine Stewardship Council (MSC) certification, and for farmed fish, look for the Aquaculture Stewardship Council (ASC) certification. Both are considered to be the most credible certification schemes for responsibly sourced fish by the WWF. As with other food from animals, eat fish and seafood justly to ensure that fish stocks can be shared fairly (see also Caretaking/Fish, page 116).

Other Considerations

As I write, there is a debate stirring around the place of animal foods, including meat, fish and dairy products, in modern diets. In an industrial food system, it takes 11 times more fossil fuel energy to produce animal protein than plant protein, gram for gram.[53] On a planet that is hurtling towards catastrophic climate change, the pointed finger of blame is aimed straight at animals. It's the cows' fault we are in this mess. However, while it is true that producing food from animals generally takes more from the Earth than producing food from plants, this is only part of the picture — a linear and reductive focus on individual foods, rather than a cyclical and holistic view of foodways.

Humans have been eating meat since the Pleistocene epoch (the Paleolithic Ice Age) — in other words, well over a million years. As you can imagine, the proportion of animal to plant foods has waxed and waned over such a vast time period. As early humans spread across the globe, they encountered many different ecologies where the availability of plant and animal foods varied considerably — not just from one place to another, but also from one season to the next.

When humans eventually transitioned to agrarian foodways in the beginnings of the Holocene epoch, they continued to integrate plants and animals, but the ways that meat was obtained changed appreciably from being wild and hunted, to being domesticated and farmed. Still though, average intakes of meat in early agrarian groups are thought to be around 5–10 kilograms a year — it was eaten around once a week, with more only during festivities.[54] Today, average meat intakes in upper income countries like Australia and New Zealand are 110–120 kilograms — over a 10-fold increase, that has only been made possible through changing production practices to be more intensive.

Rather than integrating animals sustainably and benefitting from the recycling of nutrients back into the soil and concentrating of nutrients in our bodies, we are now overcome by the system that produces them. In upper income countries, the ratio of animal to plant consumption is generally somewhere around 40:60 — probably not dissimilar to what our Paleolithic ancestors may have experienced at times.[55] But there are 7.5 billion humans on the planet now, compared to tens of thousands back then.

Trading off

To make way for so many animals and the crops to feed them, land has been cleared at a cataclysmic pace and scale and it is the main driver of deforestation and habitat loss worldwide. All counted, around three-quarters of agricultural land and nearly one-third of ice-free land on Earth is dedicated to this meaty pursuit.[56] At a time when humanity is already warming the planet's atmosphere with unprecedented amounts of greenhouse gases, the loss of trees that draw carbon back to the Earth is not insignificant. Today, this level drastically overshoots the Earth's regenerative capacity. And yet it continues.

Every year, over 1.4 billion pigs, 500 million sheep, 300 million cows and 50 billion chickens are slaughtered for their meat.[4][57] Producing such enormous numbers cheaply, necessitates that this model must operate intensively — where animals are confined to depressingly cramped, miserable living conditions, and are prevented from expressing their natural behaviours, for example, perching, scratching, dust bathing and preening

---

4   This excludes male chicks and 'unproductive' hens from egg production.

in chickens, and exploratory play behaviours in other young animals.

To fit this model, the animals themselves are selectively bred for production efficiencies — to grow ever-faster and produce the most amount of meat, milk or eggs possible. For example, in chickens raised for meat (broilers), lameness is already apparent in the short six weeks it takes to reach their target slaughter size. This causes discomfort and fractures in bones and joints, which are not adapted to support such rapid growth.[58] When naturally inquisitive rooting animals like pigs are kept in cramped conditions, they bare their frustration by biting their fellow inmates' tails. Rather than providing more space (which would sacrifice productivity efficiencies), the solution in this intensive model is to dock the pigs' tails in infancy.

Crowding animals (and fish in the case of aquaculture) into confined spaces, also brings a greater risk of disease. Here, rather than providing more space, the remedy seems to be to use preventative antibiotics to keep any emerging infections in check. Antibiotics also have the added benefit, from a productivity perspective, of working as growth promoters in some animals, including cattle and pigs (although this practice is banned in some places).[5] The use of nontherapeutic antibiotics in animal agriculture far exceeds use in human medicine and is driving the emergence and spread of antibiotic-resistant bacteria.[59] We can start to see how every decision made to maximise profit, trades off against the well-being of the animals, people and the Earth as a whole. Yet these true costs remain largely hidden.

There are now lots of humans eating lots of animals, far more than the Earth can sustain. To maintain current levels of eating animal foods, we already extract natural resources from the Earth faster than they can be replenished, and we are spilling vast quantities of warming greenhouse gases into a planet that is already on fire. This alone ought to be enough for us to reconsider this carnivorism of the Earth.

---

5   Antibiotics may also promote weight gain in humans by changing the gut microbiome, but more studies are needed to understand this better.[60]

Reconciling

The Earth has enough in her to provide everyone around 100 g red meat, 200 g poultry, 2–3 eggs, and 200 g fish a week, and 250 ml milk or dairy products a day.[61] Or, more simply, 1–2 servings of animal foods each day. This is about half of the average amount currently eaten in upper income countries (some people eat a lot more, others a lot less).[62] However, in the transition to more plant-based foodways, we should not lose sight of the bigger picture — focusing on plants, just like focusing on animals, can be reductive.

Going '*plant-based*' can mean all manner of things and is not in itself a remedy to issues that stem from the human–nature rift associated with the industrial food system. For example, eating mostly highly refined grain products, that have been produced using large amounts of polluting fossil-fuel-based agrochemicals, packaged in plastic and shipped thousands of miles to the table, is plant-based. But it is not nourishing, nor is it sustainable, and it does nothing to heal the rift.[63] A food system that works with nature in sustainable ways will look considerably different from the one we have now.

Plants *and animals* can be part of foodways that strengthen human–Earth relations. This integrative approach is known as *agroecology*. It is an art and science that is grounded in Indigenous worldviews and practices that use little to no agrochemicals, conserve nutrients, minimize waste and return what is left back to the Earth. This is already the way of three-quarters of the 1.5 billion smallholders, family farmers, and Indigenous peoples that produce over half the world's food.[64] Agroecological foodways have been woven over many generations, bounded only by nature and community, rather than making someone somewhere lots of money.

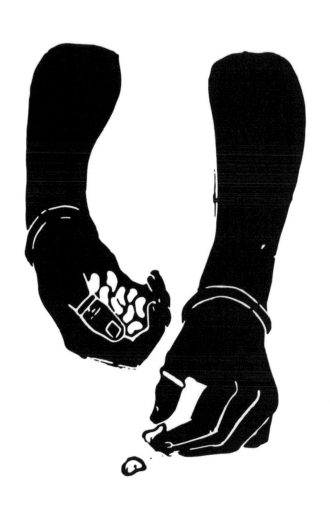

Chapter 4

PREPARE

A baby is one of a boundless array of possibilities that is brought into being by the foodways of their ancestors and parents. There is groundwork that is to be done in this preparatory time around conception — awakening fertility and renewing opportunities to connect with our bodies and appreciate fully our power to shape the future through our foodgetting.

Upbringing

Since the discovery of DNA, scientists thought that we were predetermined by the genetic blueprint from our parents. It wasn't that no attention was paid to how we are shaped by our surroundings and the life we lead, but rather, it was thought that these 'outside' factors affect us after we are born, and that their influence ends when we die. In other words, there was no sense of impermanence. It was thought that the effect of nurture was superficial — not something that could fundamentally change who we are physically, or behaviourally. However, in recent decades, this view has been turned on its head. We now have concrete evidence that our biology is inescapably shaped by our upbringing and that this embodiment starts long before we are even conceived.

The body's preparation for conception begins with gametogenesis — the creation of egg and sperm cells which eventually fuse and form the embryo. In the case of eggs, gametogenesis begins very early on in pregnancy — not your pregnancy, but your mother's pregnancy. That is, the egg that made you was created when your mother was in your grandmother's womb. And if you are pregnant with a girl, within her are the eggs that may one day become your grandchildren.[65] So much of what your grandmother experienced in her life, what your mother experienced in hers, and what you experienced in early life, is woven into you, shaping who you are today. And you are just one of many possibilities that could emerge from the set of genes you were given. If you are wondering how this can be possible, the simplest way to explain it is that the way genes are

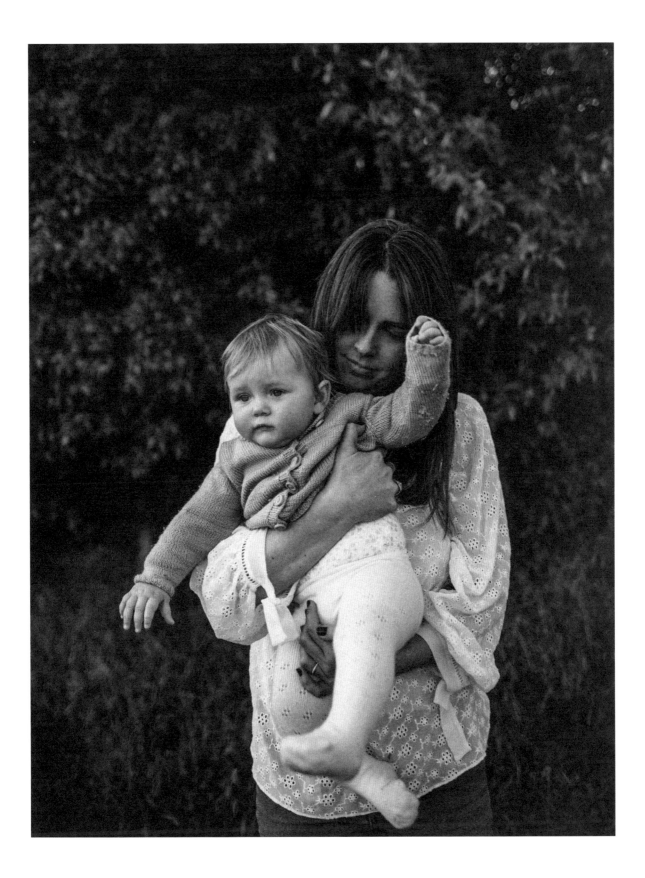

read is changeable by context, even if the genes are not themselves changed.

All of the cells in a developing embryo have the potential to turn into the many kinds of cells that are needed to grow a baby — a process known as cell differentiation. Embryonic germ cells contain a full set of genes, which can be turned on or off to varying degrees, much like a dimmer switch. Cells which differentiate into brain cells contain all the same genes, it's just that some of these are turned on and others turned off. Bone cells will have different genes turned on and others turned off, and so on. To continue this analogy, think of the controller of the dimmer switch as the context or environment. The environment affects how the dimmer switch operates and how the genes are read. This context is ever present. Even before implantation, the embryo is encircled by a special and unique fluid that is a microcosm of the outside world — a cocoon that continually provides signals that change the way the embryo develops.[66]

The environment could include the presence or absence of certain nutrients, hormones, toxins, or perhaps other genes. Yet, while we know that certain nutrients, such as folate and choline, are particularly important for turning on key genes that support development (see also Folate, page 271), there is so much we don't know about the intricacies of the inner workings of these dimmer switches. We can, however, at least appreciate that life is undoubtedly rich with potential. And although the past is beyond our control, we do have a hand in our future and that of the generations that follow.

Certain times in life are especially influential in shaping lifelong development and this is notably true of the pre- and peripartum periods — once a gene and environment interact to produce a certain outcome, that outcome persists in all cell cycles that follow (even if the environment changes in future).[67] Indeed, long before conception even takes place, nourishing foodways positively affect a mother's and baby's health during pregnancy. Studies show that *at least* three years before, high intakes of fresh fruit and vegetables, nuts, pulses and fish, significantly reduce a woman's risk in pregnancy of developing gestational diabetes, high blood pressure and preterm birth.[68]

Groundwork

Fertility is widely regarded as a window into whole-body well-being.[69] And there is very strong evidence that nourishing foodways have a positive effect on a couple's fertility and a baby's long-term health. For example, a study following over 17,500 women for eight years found that eating well lowered the risk of infertility caused by ovulatory issues by two-thirds.[70] In men, higher fruit and vegetable intakes have been linked to improved chances of success with assisted conception treatment.[71]

The body relies on nourishment to orchestrate the rhythmical hormones of menstruation and pregnancy, and to provide the sustenance to enable the growth of a whole new being. During pregnancy, the increase in demand for some nutrients is so great that to provide enough involves tapping into a mother's nutritional reserves, some of which are amassed before conception takes place. For example, towards the end of pregnancy, pre-laid maternal fat stores are tapped into to supply ample fats for a baby's rapidly growing brain.[72]

Yet, it is not uncommon for couples to go into pregnancy nutritionally underprepared. There are many reasons for this. Pregnancies are not always planned, and even when couples knowingly enter this preparatory space, there are many elements of past lifeways that can affect fertility. Men may also not realise the equal role they play in cultivating a healthful environment for pregnancy to happen.

For women who have recently taken hormonal contraceptives, this may have impacted their nutritional readiness by affecting their body's handling of nutrients. Unfortunately, however, this can manifest in different ways from person to person. For example, hormonal contraceptives can affect the absorption or excretion of nutrients, reduce the conversion of nutrients into bioactive forms, or alter nutrient metabolism by affecting hormonal balance.[73] They may reduce the levels of many vitamins and minerals, including the B complex, in particular folate and B12, but they can also improve iron stores, as oestrogen increases the body's absorption of iron and blood losses are reduced as well.[74]

For women who have been pregnant before, their body may have been depleted and the chance of this increases with each pregnancy.[75] Closely spaced pregnancies can exacerbate depletion and increase the risk of developing deficiencies, as there is less time for recuperation between birth cycles.[76] For women who have breastfed or are breastfeeding while trying to conceive or when pregnant, this places a greater nutritional demand on a woman than the pregnancy itself.[77] While this is not a reason to stop breastfeeding, it should not be overlooked when thinking about preparedness.

For women with prolonged depletion of nutritional stores, anaemia can develop. Anaemia is a deficiency in one or more nutrients, including iron, B12 and folate, and is a state when nutrient levels can't match a body's needs to function properly. Anaemia is very common in women of reproductive age. It can be caused by limited foodways and/or some of the reasons already discussed. But there are also other reasons why anaemia is more prevalent now than in times past. Notably, women today generally have far fewer pregnancies — menstruating as much as 10 times more across their reproductive lifetimes.[78] This increased blood loss takes a toll on the body, increasing the need for blood-building nutrients from foods, far beyond what our ancestors would have required.

If any of these factors feel relevant to you, consider your previous experiences and the impacts these may have had on your nutritional health. As well, if you already have a child(ren), do not underestimate the extra physical demands that raising them places on your body. Have you had enough time, care and nourishment to recover from past pregnancies, births and experiences as a mother? Some restoration of nutrition status can occur quickly, whereas in other cases it can take time.

As you contemplate the journey ahead, I invite you to hold space in this time before conception to reflect on how together, you and your partner can weave nourishing foodways and restore depletions that may be present. This is the time for groundwork — where the soil is prepared from which the seeds of a new baby and a new mother will grow.

Awakening Fertility

For some couples, the path to conception can be long and hard. Estimates suggest that around one in six experience difficulties conceiving. Infertility — the inability to conceive after a year or more of regular unprotected sex — is affecting more and more couples. And while the cause of infertility may be determined through investigations, for many, the struggle to conceive can go unexplained.[79] Couples experiencing infertility, whether the cause is known or not, may need support to conceive through assisted conception treatment, such as in vitro fertilisation (IVF). There are several conditions that are commonly related to infertility in women, including polycystic ovary syndrome, endometriosis and fibroids, as well as certain lifestyle factors in men.

Polycystic Ovary Syndrome

Polycystic Ovary Syndrome (PCOS) is very common, affecting around one in ten women of childbearing age. With PCOS, high levels of sex hormones including testosterone (known as *hyperandrogenism*) lead to symptoms of hormonal imbalance, such as acne and facial hair. Cysts also develop on the ovaries, which can be seen with ultrasound imaging. Due to these hormonal changes, PCOS significantly disrupts the rhythm of menstruation and ovulation, and it is the leading cause of anovulatory infertility (when the body does not ovulate).

The cause of PCOS is unclear and may stretch as far back to a baby's experience in the womb.[80] There is a connection with vitamin D — women with PCOS are more likely to be deficient in this nutrient.[81] A study of women with PCOS found that those with healthy vitamin D levels had thicker endometria and a better chance of conceiving.[82]

Blood sugar control also seems key. Insulin stimulates the production of sex hormones and insulin resistance is a common (but not universal) feature of PCOS. However, whether insulin resistance is a cause of or is caused by PCOS is a chicken or egg question that scientists don't have an answer to yet.

About half of women with PCOS have good blood sugar control but may still experience inflammation and oxidative stress.[83] Inflammation is a normal response by the immune system to protect against invading pathogens. However, in the absence of any infection, a chronic, low-grade inflammation has been connected to many chronic diseases including cardiovascular disease, type 2 diabetes and several cancers.[84] Both inflammation and oxidative stress also exacerbate the hormonal imbalances associated with PCOS, and conversely, increased levels of sex hormones promote inflammation and oxidative stress. In other words, a self-perpetuating cycle follows. Nourishing foodways can be effective in reducing inflammation and oxidative stress, and calming the raised blood sugar levels associated with PCOS, and are essential to restore fertility in women affected by this condition.[85]

Endometriosis

Menstruation is a cycle of tissue injury and repair. When this cycle goes awry, endometrial tissue can spread outside the uterus and create lesions, which continue to be influenced by menstrual hormones. This means that during each menstrual cycle the lesions can bleed, causing inflammation and fibrosis in nearby tissues. Endometriosis often enters the ovaries where it can also affect the ovarian egg reserve. It can be an incredibly painful experience and, unfortunately, endometriosis is a progressive disease, worsening over time.

Endometriosis affects around one in ten women of reproductive age.[86] Not all women with endometriosis experience infertility but it is more common in women with infertility — with one in three affected. Many women with infertility and endometriosis (which may or may not be related) require assisted conception treatment to get pregnant.[87] A process known as 'retrograde menstruation' is often given as the cause of endometriosis. This is where menstrual tissue flows backwards into the fallopian tubes and from there beyond the uterine walls. However, retrograde menstruation happens in nine out of ten women, most of whom do not develop endometriosis, so there are clearly other factors at play.[88]

New research points to a possible link between endometriosis and gut health, as women affected are two to three times more likely to experience irritable bowel syndrome (IBS) than those without.[89] Early work with gluten-free eating has shown strong positive results in reducing pain symptoms.[90] A study that followed over 80,000 women for twenty years found that eating red meat (processed or unprocessed) more than once a week also increased the risk of endometriosis.[91, 92] There is also a connection between endometriosis progression and inflammation and oxidative stress, as there is with PCOS.

Fibroids

Benign uterine tumours, called fibroids (or leiomyomas), are extremely common — more than half of women develop them by the time they reach fifty.[93] It is unclear precisely what causes fibroids, though there are some known risk factors, including hormonal disruptions, certain ethnicities, early onset periods (before 10 years of age), caffeine and/or alcohol consumption, and several genes. Fibroids can be associated with infertility and early pregnancy loss, however, plenty of women find they don't interfere at all, and there are treatment options available.[94] Fibroids are often an underlying cause of anaemia, including iron deficiency, in women in their thirties and forties.[95]

Infertility in Men

Over the past 40 years, a worldwide collapse in male fertility has emerged. Estimates suggest that male fertility has declined by at least half over this

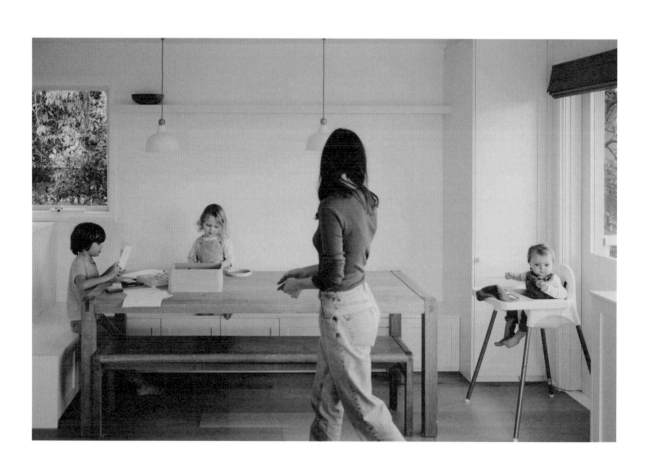

time period.[96] Statistics differ from place to place, but generally a third to half of infertility cases are ascribed to male factors, amounting to 30 million men.[97] There are myriad causes and contributors to male infertility, which are usually grouped into genetic, developmental (early life experiences), and lifestyle factors, of which foodways are a critical part. High intakes of processed meats, industrial trans fats, sugary drinks and caffeine are all connected to reduced sperm quality and/or quantity.[98] On the other hand, more essential fats, including those from fish, and unsprayed fruit and vegetables are shown to improve fertility outcomes in men.[99]

Nourishing Foundations

Foodways that awaken fertility are the same as those that are nourishing in this time before and around conception — motherfood is food for life. In this time of grounding, let us explore two areas that may centre our attention on weaving healthful practices by bringing balance to the stream of nourishment we give our bodies and by minimising hormonal disruptions.

Bringing Balance

Balanced blood sugar levels are an important determinant of ovulatory function and fertility in all women.[100] When carbohydrate-containing foods are eaten, they are digested and absorbed and released into the blood as sugar — glucose. It is important that blood sugar levels do not fluctuate wildly because, while the brain needs a steady supply of glucose for energy, routinely high blood sugar levels can cause tissue damage.

When glucose enters the bloodstream, the pancreas ordinarily secretes a hormone called insulin to clear the sugar from the blood; either making it available for immediate energy use or storing it for later in the liver and muscles. However, regularly eating large amounts of foods or drinks containing rapidly absorbed carbohydrates, such as sugary drinks and fruit juices, chocolate, confectionery, baked goods (cakes, biscuits, etc.), refined grains (white rice), is not something the body is used to in an evolutionary sense.[101] This can put a lot of pressure on the pancreas to keep up with bringing sugar levels down and can eventually lead to a condition called insulin resistance.

Insulin resistance is when insulin doesn't work effectively in clearing sugar from the blood. The pancreas tries to compensate by releasing more and more insulin, however, there are limits to how much the body can respond in this way. Eventually, blood sugar levels remain higher than are healthy. Insulin resistance is particularly problematic for fertility as it disrupts hormonal rhythms by promoting testosterone production.

Several studies have found a link between higher intakes of rapidly absorbed carbohydrates and reduced fertility, including increased odds of anovulation, a lower number of eggs successfully collected, and reduced success overall with IVF.[102, 103] For example, one study that followed the conception journey of more than 18,000 healthy women found that those who ate more carbohydrates, especially sources that were more rapidly absorbed, had nearly twice the risk of ovulatory infertility than those who ate fewer carbohydrates of better quality.[104]

Choosing slow-release, whole food sources of carbohydrates such as whole grains and fruit, and pulses in place of quick-release added sugars, highly processed grains and grain-based products, and spreading them across the day, will support the body to effectively handle the sugars from food. Also, when foods containing essential and plant-based fats and proteins are enjoyed alongside foods containing carbohydrates, these can further calm the release of sugar into the blood. A study with 18,555 women found that those who ate more plant foods containing protein, like pulses and nuts, had 50 per cent lower risk of experiencing ovulatory infertility.[105]

Disrupting Chemicals

The hormonal system, otherwise known as the endocrine system, includes various glands such as the thyroid, adrenal and pituitary, which release signals that direct body functions and behaviour. Hormone disrupting chemicals interfere with this system by blocking or mimicking hormones and changing the way the body functions. It is very concerning that there are hundreds, if not more than a thousand, hormone disrupting chemicals that we are routinely exposed to in modern life.[106, 107] Many of these chemicals are found in everyday food packaging, pesticides and animal feeds — all of which contaminate the food we eat. This is particularly problematic when foods are heated or cooled in packaging and dinnerware, as temperature changes promote the leaching of chemicals.

For a while at least, these chemicals were not thought to pose a significant health threat in the minute amounts that they are consumed. However, research is mounting that strongly challenges this presumption. Hormone disrupting chemicals are now recognised as a serious and urgent threat to public health by the World Health Organization and the International Federation of Gynaecology and Obstetrics.[108]

Hormone disrupting chemicals can influence health throughout life, including reducing fertility in men and women, and success with IVF.[109] Scientists have known since the late seventies that sperm are particularly sensitive to oxidative damage — men who have higher levels of hormone disrupting chemicals in their urine also appear to have reduced sperm quality and go on to have reduced odds of successfully conceiving with IVF.[110] During pregnancy, these chemicals can affect a woman's metabolism, promoting weight gain and influencing insulin resistance, both of which have flow on effects to a baby's development. Research also shows that the placenta is not an effective buffer of hormone disrupting chemicals, allowing them to pass freely into cord blood, amniotic fluid and the baby. Later on, they also transfer into breast milk. Compared with adults, babies and children have a significantly reduced capacity to deal with these chemicals.[111]

Most of the research investigating the effects of hormone disrupting chemicals on women and babies has focused on Bisphenol-A (BPA) and phthalates, so I have covered these below. However, it is important to note that there are many more hormone-disrupting chemicals in our foodways that we are only just starting to learn about.

Bisphenol-A

Bisphenol-A (BPA) is an industrial chemical that has been in use since the sixties. It was the first synthetic oestrogen produced and it is widespread in plastic food and drink packaging, plastic dinnerware, and in the resin lining on some cans and bottle tops. It may also be used in dental sealants. As much as 90 per cent of the BPA people are exposed to comes from packaged foods.[112] In response to growing concerns around the ill-effects of BPA, the chemical was banned in plastic baby bottles in Europe in 2011, however, its use elsewhere is as widespread as ever. Some companies have voluntarily removed BPA from their food and drink packaging, however, replacements such as Bisphenol-S (BPS) and Bisphenol-F (BPF) have been found to have similar, if not worse, health effects than BPA.[113]

Phthalates

Phthalates are synthetic plasticisers and are mainly found in personal care products including cosmetics, but also pesticides and food packaging. Packaged animal products and fried or rich takeaway foods are major sources of phthalates, because fats promote the leaching of phthalates from packaging. Animal studies have shown that phthalates affect egg development and women with endometriosis have been found to have higher levels of these compounds, suggesting a link.[114] In men, phthalates have been found to cause DNA damage in sperm.

When thinking about ways of reducing exposure to hormone disrupting chemicals, the best approach to take is one of avoidance and minimisation, rather than substitution, i.e. looking for packaging without BPA, given the continued questions around the unknown safety of alternatives. However, it can be very difficult to avoid plastic food packaging and other sources of hormone-disrupting chemicals.

A recent US study found people who ate more highly processed packaged products had higher levels of hormone-disrupting chemicals in their pee, so it will help to lessen their use.[115] However, even when minimising the amount of highly processed products, many whole foods such as beans, lentils, cooked tomatoes and whole grains often come in cans or plastic packaging. Even so, research shows that reducing exposure where possible is worthwhile and pays off remarkably quickly. A study where participants switched to fresh, organic foods, in plastic-free packaging and non-plastic containers found that the levels of hormone-disrupting chemicals in pee dropped between 53 per cent and 66 per cent in only three days.[116]

Ways to reduce exposure to hormone-disrupting chemicals
— Enjoy mostly seasonal, fresh (especially unsprayed), unpackaged foods
— Try bulk food stores that decant goods into paper or fabric bags
— Choose foods and drinks packaged in uncoated paper/cardboard or glass over plastic or cans
— Avoid cooking and storing foods in plastic packaging
— Use loose leaf teas (many tea bags contain plastic) or a French press or drip coffee in place of plastic 'coffee pod' type products
— Avoid eating partially charred or burned foods[6]
— Choose stainless steel, cast iron, ceramic or enamelware cooking and storage equipment, and beeswax wraps or similar for storage, and phase out any non-stick cookware[7], and plastic utensils and storage containers

---

6   Foods that are burned through grilling, barbecuing, toasting and frying form hormone disrupting chemicals called 'advanced glycation end-products' (AGEs).[117]
7   Non-stick cookware may contain polyfluoroalkyl (PFAS), a hormone disrupting chemical which has been linked to reduced birthweight.[118]

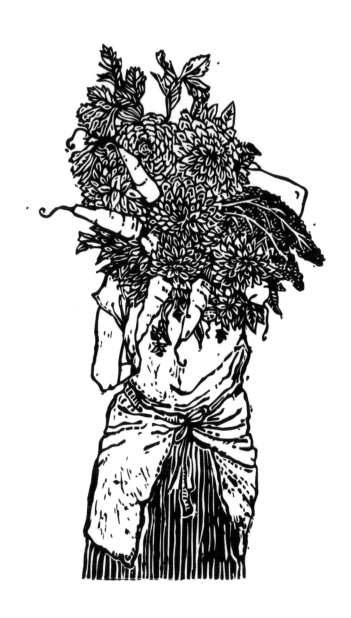

Chapter 5

SENSE

Pregnancy is an exceptional time — a season in a woman's life when she experiences a connection that, outside of the womb of her own mother, transcends anything she encounters her entire life. The umbilical cord physically ties her to her baby, and it is through this ancient braid that nourishment is shared. Pregnancy offers a unique window to witness embodiment — where a woman grows outwardly and inwardly and, through doing so, experiences how her foodways become her and a whole new being.

Lifegiving

Your body is powerful — a lifeforce. In spite of all it may have taken to get you to this point of conception, trust in your body. Be reassured that your body knows what to do and prepare to be amazed by it. Already at three to seven weeks after your last menstruation (one to five weeks after conception) — before you may have even realised you were pregnant — the beginnings of your baby's organs have emerged.

In just 12 weeks, your placenta will have formed — a wholly new organ that will be the songsmith that writes the song of your baby.[119] Many traditional cultures honour the nurturing role of the placenta by describing it as a sister, mother, grandmother or as a protective covering, and take care with its surrender.[120] For example, in Māori culture, the word for land and placenta are the same — *whenua*. After birth, it is traditional practice for the placenta to be buried, returning it to the Earth (whenua to whenua) — the place from which a mother is from.

Biologically speaking, your placenta is, in fact, the same sex as your baby. She or he will take on the functions of the lungs, gut, kidneys and liver — cycling nourishment to your baby and waste away and producing the hormones that establish the rhythm and pace of your pregnancy. At this time, your body will intuitively shift the handling of nourishment to ensure it provides enough to sustain your placenta, your baby and your own body.

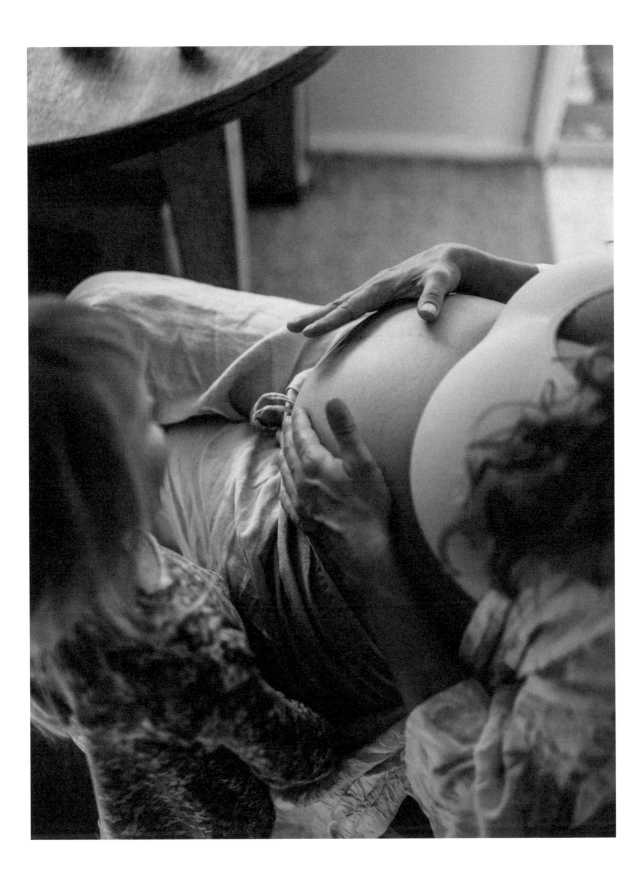

There are various ways you do this, including absorbing more nutrients from the food you ordinarily eat, recycling nutrients more efficiently and drawing upon your own reserves to make up any dietary shortfalls.

These economies mean that, during pregnancy, you need very little extra energy from your foodways — probably no more than an extra 10 per cent energy, in the third trimester only.[121] Even so, growing a baby is no mean feat. And while your body knows all of this intuitively, you can support this lifegiving work through your foodways by noticing what your body is experiencing and eating nourishing foods that feel good for you during this transitionary season.

Sensemaking

Preparing for and experiencing pregnancy and birth tunes us into our bodies in ways that we may not ordinarily experience. Opportunities emerge to observe the cycle of menstruation and notice signs of fertility, attend to changeable food preferences and gut rhythms, experience growing tummies and birthing babies, and so much more. In many ways, pregnancy is a time abounding with possibilities to reconnect with ourselves and marvel at the wonder of it all.

Morning Sickness

As you come to know your pregnant self, one of the first things you may notice is profound changes in your relationship with food. Your food preferences may shift, and you may also experience uncomfortable waves of nausea or even vomit. These feelings usually emerge relatively early on, often around week five, when the embryo is forming. They commonly arc to peak somewhere in weeks eight to twelve, and then wane thereafter.[122] This experience is often referred to as *morning sickness*, though you may notice these feelings at any time of day.

Morning sickness is experienced on a spectrum. For less than 1 per cent of women, it can be prolonged and incredibly debilitating. Excessive vomiting (more than three times a day) is known as *hyperemesis gravidarum*. At this extreme, morning sickness is potentially life-threatening. Hospital admission is usually required to manage dehydration, pain, gut changes, nutritional deficiencies and other related metabolic and/or neurological issues.

Wherever you are on the morning sickness spectrum, it can cast a huge shadow over your pregnancy and steal some enjoyment of the experience. Understanding why morning sickness is so common may provide some comfort in what can otherwise be a trying time.[123, 124] Scientists have long debated this. The prevailing view is that morning sickness is incidental and serves no purpose – that these happenings are merely an unpleasant side effect of the extreme hormonal shifts that happen in early pregnancy. However, there is little to substantiate this idea and, indeed, recent studies have provided evidence to counter it.[125]

An alternative school of thought is that morning sickness is an *inner knowing* that protects a woman during a particularly sensitive phase of pregnancy. It is during the first trimester that the embryo forms limbs and major organ systems. This is a risky time when toxins may cause lasting damage to the rapidly dividing embryonic cells. It is also a time when the immune system changes to allow for a baby which is half 'foreign' genetic material. By avoiding or purging toxic compounds or pathogens, morning sickness makes good sense from an evolutionary standpoint.[126, 127] In support of a protective role is a genetic link — if your mother experienced hyperemesis gravidarum carrying you, then you are three times more likely to experience it. If your sister experienced hyperemesis gravidarum, then you are 17 times more likely to.[128]

Practices and remedies to manage morning sickness

Though morning sickness is common in pregnancy, there is no reason to suffer through this time. In the first instance, there are some practices and

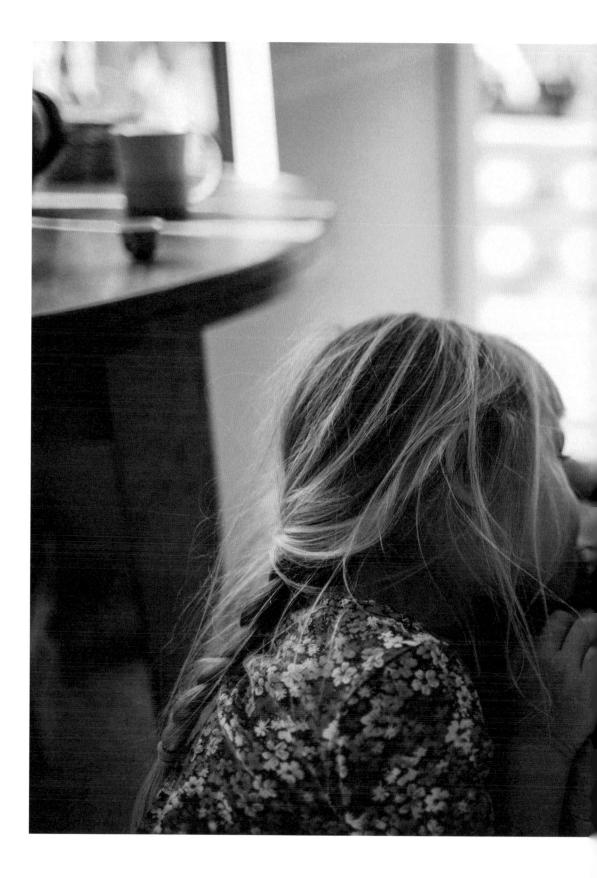

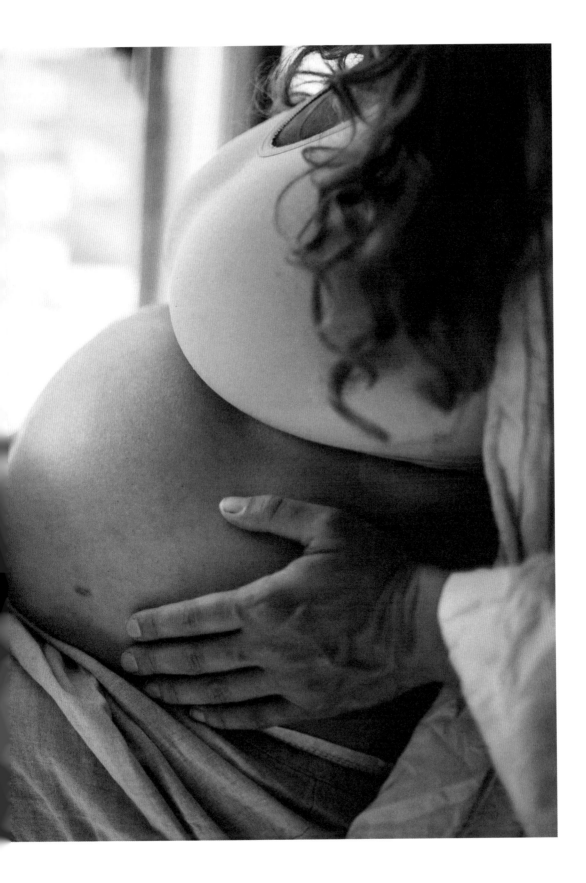

home remedies you can try that may alleviate discomfort. If you feel these are not enough and your well-being is affected speak with your doctor. Early treatment, including with pregnancy-safe anti-sickness medications, may help prevent morning sickness worsening over time.

Listen to your body: Try to avoid foods or smells that you find trigger or worsen your morning sickness, which may include rich or acidic dishes. It is often the case that we prefer simple, bland foods when we feel nauseous, such as plain crackers or dry toast (try adapting Whole Wheat Crackers and Dulse with Za'atar, page 240). Eat simply when you feel you need to and work in more flavourful, nourishing foods at a time of day when you notice your body is more receptive.

Eat little and often: When our blood sugar levels are low or drop suddenly, this can exacerbate feelings of nausea. When able to, eat small amounts regularly throughout the day to keep blood-sugar levels up. A small snack by your bed can also be a good idea before you get up for the day. Choose whole-grain foods and unsweetened drinks to avoid the surges in blood sugar that come with refined sugars and starches. Meals or snacks that are higher in protein may also help, like a handful of nuts or hard-boiled egg.

Replenish fluids and body salts: Keeping yourself hydrated is essential, especially when you are not managing much in the way of food. Cold sparkling water or ice blocks (try Ginger Tea and Melon Ice Blocks, page 236) may bring some extra reprieve beyond plain water. If you are vomiting regularly, replacing electrolytes is also important. Over the counter electrolyte drinks are available or sipping on a nourishing broth would also help (try Miso, Ginger and Barley Broth with Wilted Greens, page 205). Keep an eye on your pee. It should be clear and colourless or pale yellow. After your first morning pee, cloudy yellow is a sign your body needs more water. Dark yellow, orange or brown suggests dehydration and you should speak with your doctor about quick and safe replenishment.

Rest and recuperate: Pregnancy can be tiring, which can intensify feelings of nausea. Call on your partner, family or friends to help cook your foods and/or offload some of your burdens and bring some respite. If possible, shift your commitments around so that you are not busy when you are feeling unwell. Rest and move as much as feels good for you.

GINGER ROOT

Ginger (*Zingiber officinale*) is a rhizome (an enlarged underground stem) native to tropical India. Known as stem ginger when it is young, research shows it to be effective in reducing pregnancy-related nausea, but not necessarily vomiting. Ginger has no known side effects, and it is recommended by the main colleges of obstetrics and gynaecology.[129, 130]

The dosage of dried ginger that has been shown to be effective is 1 gram spread throughout the day in three or four doses for at least four days (note that 1 gram dried ginger is equal to around 6 grams fresh). Use ginger liberally in your cooking and/or sip ginger tea throughout the day to see if it offers some reprieve. There are several recipes in this book that make use of ginger. Of note are the Gingernut Biscuits with Oats and Dried Apricots (page 245), which are super to nibble on when you can't manage much by way of a full meal.

FRESH GINGER TEA

All seasons

Serves *1*
Time *10 minutes*

A knob of fresh ginger root, scrubbed and thinly sliced or grated (see Note below)
Optional:
Lemon slices or a squeeze of half a lemon
1 star anise
Honey, maple syrup or another sweetener, to taste

Steep the ginger (with optional ingredients if desired) for 5 to 10 minutes in boiled water and drain.

A larger pot can be made and sipped throughout the day, by increasing the amount of water and ginger.

> *NOTE*
> *You can use an ordinary grater, or a Japanese grater known as an oroshigane, which grates the ginger very finely.*

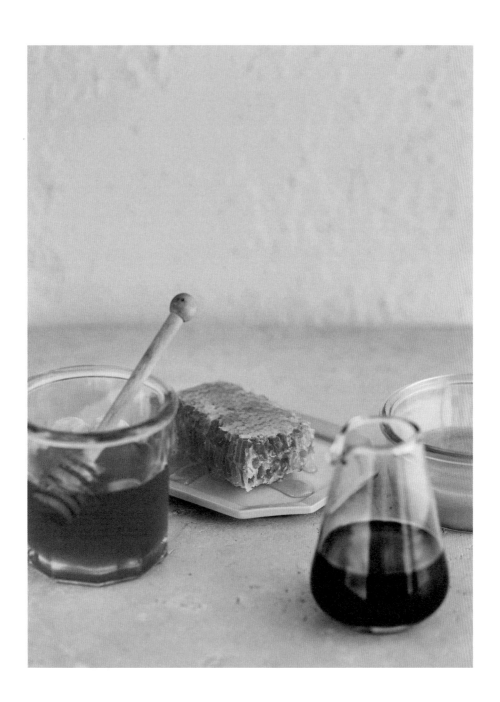

Food Cravings

As the unpleasantness of morning sickness subsides, you may notice the emergence of strong urges for particular foods. Like morning sickness, food cravings often follow an arc pattern in their intensity, but in this case, the peak generally happens in the second trimester and then falls away thereafter.[131] There is huge variety in the foods that women crave within, but especially across, cultures. It is possible that cravings are another example of *inner knowing* — where food preferences adjust to meet nutritional needs, but there is little evidence that supports this.

Food cravings also fall on a spectrum where at the extreme (though not uncommon) end, a woman may have a strong desire to eat non-food items, such as earth, paper or chalk. The word to describe this practice, *pica*, comes from the Latin *pica-pica*, meaning magpie — a bird known for gathering a wide variety of random objects to build their nests. Researchers have suggested it is possible that pica may provide protection by reducing the absorption of harmful toxins and/or strengthening the gut lining.[132] Indeed, in some African cultures, pica is socially accepted as it is believed to confer benefits to a woman during pregnancy.[133] However, unlike food cravings, non-food items may contain toxic compounds or parasites, and it is best not to act on these inclinations, however strong they are.

Gut Changes

During pregnancy you may observe changes to the way that food passes through your body and discomfort may arise. Multiple happenings contribute to this. Much of the digestive tract is muscle that works to pulse food along from one end to the other. Pregnancy hormones relax these muscles and, in doing so, slow the movement of food through your gut. While the upside of this is that more nourishment can be absorbed, the downside is that food hangs around for longer, sometimes leading to reflux or constipation. Your uterus also expands. This takes up space that is ordinarily home to your digestive system. And there are changes to the gut microbiota, which may come into play as well. Noticing these changes arms you with ways of responding and ensures you can be as comfortable as possible.

Reflux

There is a valve that sits where the oesophagus (food pipe) meets the stomach. Usually, this valve prevents food moving backwards, however, pregnancy hormones relax its tone, making it unable to perform this role as effectively. As food also waits for longer in the stomach before moving into the intestine and there is increased upwards pressure beneath the stomach, this may cause acid to move into the oesophagus and result in tissue damage and discomfort.

Reflux has similar symptoms to heartburn but, in pregnancy, reflux is often more troublesome, as it usually lasts longer and can occur at any time of day.[134] Symptoms related to reflux include a persistent cough, chest pain, sinusitis, and an acid taste in the mouth. Pay attention to how eating practices trigger these symptoms — a food and symptom diary may help with this. Explore ways you can adapt what and how you eat to ease things. For example, you may find smaller meals more comfortable. Fluids kept to between meals can also ensure that your stomach is not overly full. Not eating too close to bedtime and keeping your head slightly elevated may encourage gravity to keep things moving down the right way.

Pregnancy-safe, aluminium-free antacids, such as calcium carbonate, may be used to neutralise stomach acid. However, it is worth noting that the absorption of folate is dependent on an acidic pH and so the use of antacids can reduce its absorption.[135]

Constipation and Diarrhoea

Constipation is very common in pregnancy, especially during the first and second trimesters. Everyone's bowel movements are different. If you notice that you are opening your bowels less often than before, experiencing difficulty passing hard stools or feel like you are not fully cleared, then there may be ways of easing things.

Fruit is especially helpful here. Drying fruit concentrates the natural compounds that aid gut motility. Prunes and prune juice are good, but also other dried fruit such as apricots, dates and figs can help. As well, gradually increasing the amounts of whole foods you eat, including coarse grains, pulses, fresh fruit and vegetables, will support digestion. Keeping hydrated is important for soft bowel movements and being active helps too. If you find these suggestions bring little or no reprieve, you may like to speak with your doctor or pharmacist about pregnancy-safe laxatives or stool softeners.

Constipation together with extra pressure from your baby in the pelvic area may also increase the risk of developing haemorrhoids. When mild, haemorrhoids can be treated with warm water baths or a cloth soaked in witch hazel. Again, speak with your doctor or pharmacist if discomfort is intense or prolonged.

Some recipes that may help with constipation
— Poached Pear and Prune Crumble with Almonds and Dark Chocolate, page 232
— Chocolate and Cashew Shake, page 239

During pregnancy, diarrhoea is generally a less common issue than constipation and bouts are usually short-lived. If you experience diarrhoea, it is important to keep hydrated (follow the same advice given for fluid replenishment with morning sickness) and practice good hygiene. When nausea and vomiting are experienced jointly with diarrhoea, a gut infection is a possibility. A high temperature makes this more likely. If diarrhoea lasts more than a day, or is very watery or bloody, it is advisable to speak with your doctor.

Gestational Diabetes

As pregnancy progresses, the body becomes increasingly resistant to insulin, so much so that towards late pregnancy, it may be half as sensitive to insulin as before.[136] This is a natural phenomenon that happens to all women during pregnancy. Insulin is a hormone with many functions, but its key role is to remove sugar (glucose) from the blood.[137] Insulin resistance results in blood-sugar levels that are higher than usual. This is helpful for the baby — glucose is the main energy source that fuels growth in the womb. However, there are concerns that if blood-sugar levels are continually too high, this aspect of pregnancy tips from being beneficial to harmful. Prolonged high blood-sugar levels can increase the risk of developing other health issues. These include pre-eclampsia, preterm delivery and c-section during pregnancy, and, in the long-term, type 1 and 2 diabetes and other metabolic disturbances. Gestational diabetes can also affect a baby's growth and long-term health.

There are several factors that can increase the risk of developing gestational diabetes including age, smoking and inactivity. Countries differ in whether and how they check for gestational diabetes. Some will first assess likelihood by screening with questions about the aforementioned risk factors. Others will routinely carry out an oral glucose-tolerance test. Whichever the approach taken, it is common to check for gestational diabetes at mid- to late-pregnancy, as this is the time when the body's resistance to insulin and blood-sugar levels are naturally at their highest.

A diagnosis of gestational diabetes can create anxiety, however, there is a lot that can be done. In the first instance, maintaining or shifting towards nourishing foodways and moving the body more are proven to be very effective and are the main approach for three-quarters of women.[138] To calm blood-sugar levels so that they are not continuously raised or regularly peaking at high levels, the emphasis is on providing nourishing whole foods, in moderate portions, spaced evenly across the day (see also Bringing Balance, page 95).

You may be encouraged to monitor your blood-sugar levels to understand their rhythm and response to any dietary and lifestyle changes. After a couple of weeks, your doctor may assess whether you need more intensive support such as medication or insulin injections. Any drug therapy will usually continue for the remainder of your pregnancy.

Caretaking

For all that pregnancy is a time of strength — a time when a woman openly reveals her lifegiving power — it is also a time of intense vulnerability, when her immune system undergoes deep and complex changes, some of which increase susceptibility to food poisoning. As one example, during pregnancy, women are 17 times more likely to get Listeriosis, which can cause complications including premature delivery or miscarriage.[139] Pregnancy is a time to take extra care to use safe and hygienic food practices to ensure the risk of contracting an infection is minimised. It is also wise to avoid those foods which are more likely to harbour the bacteria that can lead to food poisoning. See the table opposite for a guide.

Fish

Beyond concerns around food poisoning, there are additional considerations for fish due to the presence of heavy metals and pollutants, including methylmercury and polychlorinated biphenyls (PCBs). Methylmercury is neurotoxic and can cause extensive damage to the brain and nervous system. As it readily crosses the placenta, babies in the womb are especially vulnerable to its effects. The metabolites of PCBs accumulate in fatty body tissues and due to their resemblance to natural hormones, it is thought that they can disrupt thyroid hormone metabolism.[140]

Unfortunately, the advice on how much fish women can safely eat is mixed and often complex in regard to 'allowable' species and serving

	Avoid	Enjoy
Cheese	Soft ~ Uncooked soft blue-veined cheese, e.g. Gorgonzola, Danish Blue, Roquefort	Soft ~ Well-cooked soft cheeses with blue veins or mould rinds
	~ Uncooked soft mould-ripened cheese, e.g. Brie, Camembert, chèvre	~ Uncooked pasteurised soft cheese, e.g. ricotta, mascarpone, cream cheese, cottage cheese, labne
	Hard None	Semi-soft or hard ~ Hard cheese with blue veins, e.g. Stilton ~ Semi-soft or hard cheeses, e.g. Cheddar, Parmesan, feta
Eggs	~ Raw, uncooked or soft-boiled eggs, including where these are an ingredient such as mayonnaise	~ Well-cooked eggs and meringue (provided it is cooked thoroughly and is firm/hard, i.e. not sticky in the middle)
Milk	~ All unpasteurised milk products	~ Pasteurised milk products, e.g. crème fraîche, fromage frais
Pâté	~ Meat and vegetable pâtés	
Meat	~ Raw or undercooked meat, including cold cured meats, e.g. salami, chorizo	~ Well-cooked (cured or uncured) meat or poultry
Fish	~ Raw fish, smoked fish or seafood, sushi	~ Well-cooked fish, smoked fish or seafood
Misc.	Tahini, including hummus made with it (see Foods from Plants, page 40), pre-packaged salads, uncooked sprouted grains and pulses, unpasteurised fruit juice	

sizes. To be on the safe side, many women may simply avoid eating fish altogether. However, studies show that despite the risks, eating fish during pregnancy can be beneficial to a baby's development and long-term health, so it is worth clearing up what a reasonable approach is safety-wise.

Methylmercury and PCBs are so widespread in the environment that all fish embody them to some degree. However, depending on where fish fit in aquatic food webs, there are big differences in the amount of methylmercury that fish contain. Fish size is the best guide — long-lived and predatory species, such as king mackerel, marlin, shark, snapper, swordfish and larger species of tuna, are 'higher up' the food web and contain large amounts of methylmercury — these should be avoided when trying to conceive, and during pregnancy and breastfeeding.

Smaller fish like anchovies and sardines, as well as herring, mackerel, Pacific salmon and line caught freshwater trout are relatively low in methylmercury, are all rich in essential fats, and can usually be obtained from sustainable fisheries — though not all are.[141] If you would like to eat fish safely, one serving (140 grams cooked)[8] of a variety of small, sustainably caught oily fish a week, probably strikes a good balance between concerns around toxins, pollutants and sustainability, while still reaping the many health benefits that fish have to offer.[142]

Liver

From the very beginnings of pregnancy, vitamin A plays a major role in instructing cells to differentiate — to become the many different types of cells needed to create a human body. Women need more vitamin A than usual at this time to provide for the many roles that this essential nutrient performs. However, the increased need for vitamin A is only slight, and too much as well as not enough vitamin A can cause widespread ill-effects,

---

8   Note that many health organisations recommend two portions of fish a week, one of which should be oily, however, this prioritises human health over the health and sustainability of fishing practices needed to meet these recommendations (see Foods from Animals, page 77).

including birth defects (see Micronutrients, page 269). The liver is where many animals store nutrients for later use, making it a rich source of many compounds including high levels of vitamin A. Due to this, many health organisations advise against eating liver and cod liver oil and taking supplements containing vitamin A during pregnancy.

Modern life increases our exposure to vitamin A. It can be found in many highly processed products that are fortified to 'enrich' their depleted nutritional content, including some breakfast cereals and margarine. Vitamin A is also found in some supplements and topical preparations such as skin creams. Even in whole food sources, the vitamin A content of liver has (at least for some animals) increased considerably due to giving animals feed that is fortified with the vitamin.[143]

If you eat little in the way of products fortified with vitamin A and are not exposed to it from skin creams, then you may like to have liver during pregnancy, especially given its broad nutritional benefits. Waiting until the second trimester and having occasional small amounts is plenty enough. The World Health Organization has noted that 50–70 grams of cooked liver weekly or less often, poses no significant teratogenic risk.[144] But eating even less than that once a week, by grating a little (say 25 grams) frozen grass-fed liver into a stew, chilli or similar and cooking it through well, would be a simple way of significantly and safely boosting the nourishing qualities of a meal.[145] Eating small amounts of liver could be especially valuable with plant-based eating — providing a keen dose of nutrition in a small parcel of food.

Vitamin A content of liver[146]

Calf liver — 2500–3500 µg per 25 g uncooked
Poultry liver — 2500–3000 µg per 25 g uncooked
Beef liver — 1250–3750 µg per 25 g uncooked
Pork liver — 2500–3500 µg per 25 g uncooked

Food Allergens

Although allergic conditions such as asthma, hay fever, eczema and food allergies are on the rise, research suggests that avoiding common food allergens during pregnancy does not affect or reduce the chance of a baby developing a food allergy.[147]

Closing the Cycle

As your pregnancy season draws to a close and your baby's birth day beckons, I invite you to let go of expectations of what may come. No one can know what your birth experience will bring. And although releasing our minds into this haze of uncertainty may naturally bring restlessness, we can find grounding in the preparations that are undoubtedly needed to nourish yourself well through this transitionary phase.

You may be at home or away in a hospital or birth centre on the birth day, and the experience may last for days or be over in a flash. Whatever may be the case, thinking ahead and keeping a cool bag of some simple provisions (for you and your birth partner) will mean that you will not need to look far or wait for food, should you be in want of it. You may also like to fill up your ice cube trays — I found it incredibly soothing to suck on ice in the first phase of labour.

Some ideas of foods for birth
- Seasonal fruit and vegetables
- Nuts and dried fruit, e.g. dates, apricots, or a trail mix
- Muesli and milk, e.g. Zesty Oat and Almond Lightly Toasted Muesli with Apricots (page 150)
- Snack bars, e.g. Date, Hemp Seed and Almond Bars (page 246)
- Toast with nut butter, avocado, etc.
- Crackers, e.g. Whole Wheat Crackers and Dulse with Za'atar (page 240)

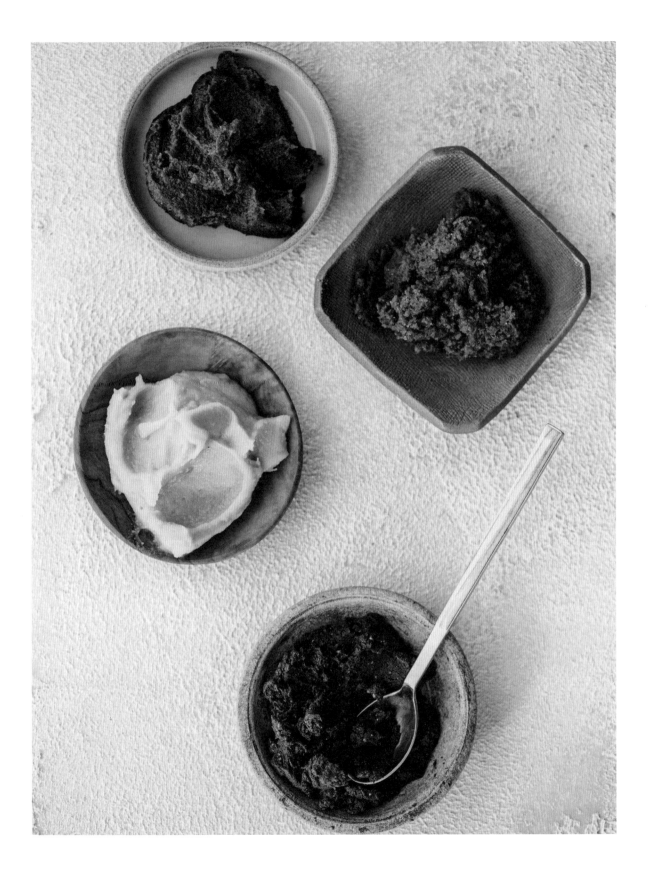

- Soup kept in an insulated flask
- Cold salad, e.g. Spelt Berry, Sunflower Seed, Apricot and Apple Pilaf with Caraway (page 173), Roast Cauliflower, Chickpea and Bulgur Salad with Ras el Hanout (page 165)
- Muffins, e.g. Sun-dried Tomato and Pesto Muffins with Pepitas (page 224), Whole Wheat Porridge Muffins with Apples and Dates (page 157)

In the newborn weeks, if not beyond, time in motherhood will bend in strange ways — slowing down and whizzing by all at the same time. Planning for this tumultuous season as best we can will go a long way in supporting your recuperation by ensuring you have nourishing foods to hand. Batch cooking wholesome meals and freezing them in portions and replenishing the pantry and cupboards so they are well stocked is worth doing. Check you have things like whole grains, pasta, quick cook and/or canned pulses, nuts, and other ingredients that bring dishes together — canned tomatoes, jars of passata, coconut milk, seasonings and so on.

Some ideas of foods to prep ahead for the newborn weeks
- Lentil, Chickpea and Brown Rice Harira (page 195)
- Quinoa, Potato and Corn Soup with Sweet Yellow Chilli (page 219)
- Coconut Yoghurt and Lemon Dahl with Sticky Jasmine Rice (page 206)
- Three Sisters Chilli (page 198)
- Pickled Onion and Puy Lentil Stew with Mashed Potato (page 215)
- Miso, Ginger and Barley Broth with Wilted Greens (add the greens when reheating) (page 205)

Beyond stocking up the freezer and store cupboard, another idea to consider is a postpartum *meal circle*, sometimes called a meal train. This is when your friends and family come together to provide a calendar of nourishment in the newborn weeks. Connecting through food in this way is a wonderful concept to support a newborn family to nourish themselves well as they transition into their new life.

Example Postpartum Meal Circle

Week	Person	Main Meal	
1	1	Roast Cauliflower, Chickpea and Bulgur Salad with Ras el Hanout	Zesty Oat and Almond Lightly Toasted Muesli with Apricots
	2	Coconut Yoghurt and Lemon Dahl with Sticky Jasmine Rice	Gingernut Biscuits with Oats and Dried Apricots
	3	Miso, Ginger and Barley Broth with Wilted Greens	Cardamom and Brown Rice Kheer with Honeyed Plums
2	4	Quinoa, Potato and Corn Soup with Sweet Yellow Chilli	Whole Wheat Porridge Muffins with Apples and Dates
	5	Black Bean and Walnut Burgers with Tomato Kasundi	Date, Hemp Seed and Almond Bars
	6	Three Sisters Chilli	Whole Wheat Crackers and Dulse with Za'atar
3	7	Pumpkin Farroto with Crispy Shredded Kale and Sage	Hazelnut, Whole Wheat and Buttermilk Pancakes with Apple
	8	Caramelised Fennel and Sun-dried Tomato Pasta with Cannellini Beans	Date and Pecan Scones with Ginger
	9	Kale, Cannellini and Farro Ribollita with Sourdough	Poached Pear and Prune Crumble with Almonds and Dark Chocolate
4	10	Lentil, Chickpea and Brown Rice Harira	Marmalade Loaf with Walnuts
	11	Pickled Onion and Puy Lentil Stew with Mashed Potato	Sun-dried Tomato and Pesto Muffins with Pepitas
	12	Squash, Sage and Baby Spinach Lasagne with Triple Tomato Lentils	Buttermilk Brownies with Cashew Caramel

A meal circle can be coordinated through a shared document online or there are websites available to help. It's a good idea to ask someone who enjoys organising to put together the meal circle on your behalf, and possibly also support by combining drop offs in the newborn days to minimise daily interruptions. On page 123 you will find an example meal circle that works with twelve people each providing a main meal and a side dish or dessert over the first month. However, this could be done with fewer people or dishes, or include some shop-bought items to make it work.

Placenta Care

The twilight of your pregnancy will bring a time to part with your placenta, and you may like to give some forethought as to what you want that to look like. A baby's first breaths open the vessels in their lungs and create space to receive blood from the placenta. This passage of air and blood marks a partial surrender of lifegiving from a mother to her baby. When possible, granting time for this sacred transition can allow much more nourishment to flow to a baby. Waiting until after the umbilical cord has stopped pulsing — usually around three minutes — may enable the transfer of somewhere around a third to half more red blood cells.[148]

As the energy of the placenta fades and the braid connecting a mother and baby stills, you may like to cut the umbilical cord. An alternative practice is a *lotus birth*, where the decision of when to let go is turned over to the baby. Lotus birth involves waiting until the cord dries and comes away and usually takes around four days.[149] If your placenta returns or stays at home with you (depending on where you birthed), you may consider returning the placenta to the Earth through burial. This is a common practice in traditional communities, often under a fruit-bearing shrub or tree in the home garden.

Placentophagy, the practice of ingesting a placenta, is often referred to as traditional practice, though there is no evidence to support this.[150, 151] Placentophagy is often promoted, though without scientific backing, to alleviate postpartum depression, improve recovery and increase breastfeeding. We should be mindful that the placenta stores toxins that are inappropriate to pass on to the baby. Whether these compounds would harm the mother when ingested is unknown. Despite the lack of evidence for benefits or harms, media reports continue to vehemently deter women from the practice. If you decide to ingest your placenta, take great care with safe handling. Preparation may involve dehydration and encapsulation, tincture, or eating it raw or cooked with herbs.

Liminality

In all your preparations for birth and the excitement that comes with these, it is easy to miss the space between — a fleeting time towards the end of pregnancy when you are called to notice the transition you are soon to make. Grant yourself the serenity to notice this liminal moment of acceptance and deep knowing. It is a space to pause and let go of your past self with gratitude, and to breathe in the days to come, as you prepare to welcome your new self. Put aside any due dates you have been prescribed and listen quietly to your body. Together, your baby and body will know the right time to initiate birthing and will be your guide on this passage into motherhood. Listen.

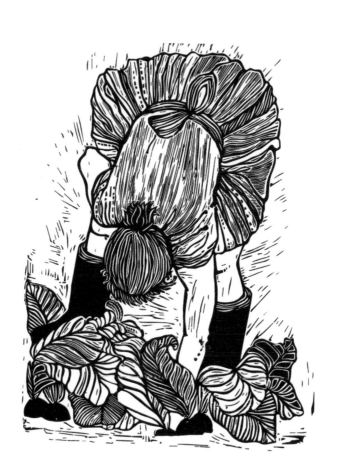

Chapter 6

RELEASE

Motherhood is an odyssey — a continuing and expansive journey where a woman is taken far from the realms of herself. A voyage that will pull her this way and that, and in doing so reveal newness — changes in herself that could only be stirred in the chaos of caring for a new life. Nurturing a mother on this passage is essential. If she is well braced by her family and community, she will have the capacity to release expectations and notice and receive the changes she discovers.

Holding a Mother

Much attention is paid to a baby. It's completely understandable that everyone wants to hold this new life that astounds us with its metamorphosis from its motherbound cocoon. In truth, however, newborn babies need only to connect with their parents — their mother, especially. Redirecting this beautiful, caregiving energy and returning attention to the mother holds both the mother and the baby, because the health and well-being of both are entirely intertwined.

Many traditional cultures recognise this interdependence and protect the newborn weeks as a sacred time of rest to restore maternal health. This time goes by different names, such as *zuo yue zi* or 'doing the month' in China. Or in Japan, *Satogaeri bunben* involves a woman travelling to her family home towards the end of pregnancy and remaining there until a couple of months after the birth.[152] Sometimes known as confinement, women surround a mother and work with intention to create a restorative space that holds for new mother–baby rhythms.

The length of time involved in *holding a mother* varies across cultures, but in general, at least a month is given over to this important work. Practices centre on providing organised support, so a mother can pause her usual day-to-day activities and refocus her attention on her baby and herself.[153] Physically, new mothers are encouraged to keep warm through hot baths or facial steams, use extra blankets and take bedrest.

The reality of life is that it is not always possible to wholly give in to this important time, and properly rest. It is unfortunate for some, that life or work commitments can intrude. Other women do not have the comfort provided by a close network of women who can extend support to a new mother. To paraphrase an old adage — *we can only do what we can, with what we have, where we are*. But be mindful of who is holding you in this time and do not be hesitant in reaching out for support or saying no to activities that can wait.

Nourishing Postpartum

Nourishing foodways are an integral part of holding a mother. Pregnancy and birth may leave you feeling physically and mentally drained. Your nutritional stores will probably be depleted, and you may have experienced blood loss. Interruptions to your sleep patterns are likely to be ongoing and your body may look and work differently right now. Be kind and gentle with yourself — recuperation and repletion will take time. Alongside tending to your baby, allow yourself the space, compassion and patience to equalise tending to yourself.

Estimates suggest that around one in five women experience depression within the first three months of giving birth, and in nearly half, negative feelings may persist beyond the first year.[154] Your postpartum foodways are key in replenishing your body's nutritional stores to nourish your body and mind. Many compounds in foods can affect our mood. For example, low iron across the peripartum period (pregnancy and nursing) is linked with depression.[155] However, feeling low can also affect the energy available to prepare nourishing meals. Anxiety or stress can also affect appetite or shift food preferences.[156] Notice how you are feeling and seek support from friends, family or healthcare professionals, if things do not feel okay.

If you breastfeed, your body will need more nourishment than ever before — even more than in pregnancy. The energy it takes to breastfeed a baby for nine months is double that needed for the whole nine months of

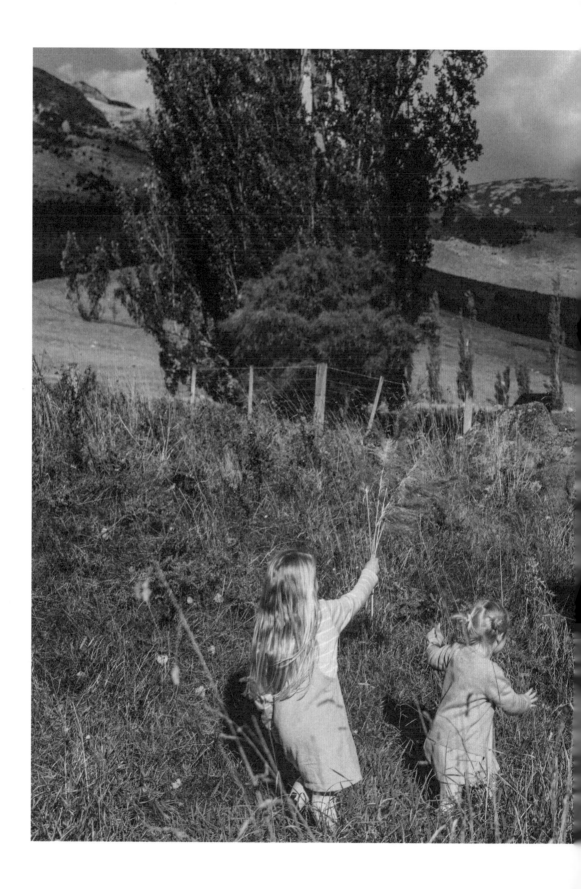

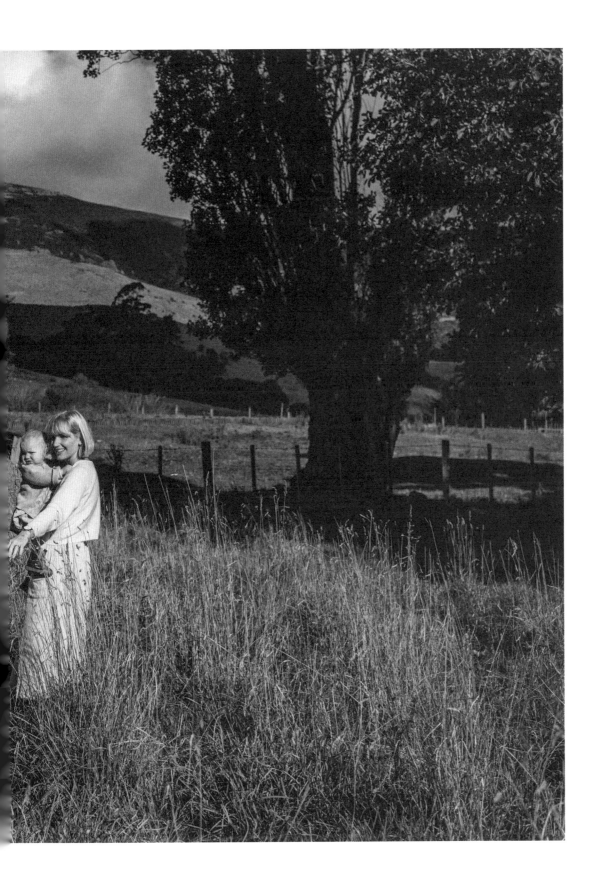

pregnancy.[157] This is even when taking into account that the reliance on breast milk lessens as an infant transitions to complementary family foods. Unless a mother is extremely depleted, her body will produce sufficient breast milk that contains all that is necessary to grow a healthy baby.

The foods to encourage in the postpartum period are no different to those that feed you well at other times — motherfood is food for life. However, your foodways may need to shift. To nourish yourself well in this season, you may need to find alternative food practices that weave well into your new life and ensure you make time to eat well. For example, you could invest in an insulated mug to keep your drink or soup hot while you tend to your baby. Or you could get key provisions delivered to your home, so that you are well supplied with staple foods. Continuing to batch cook meals and leaning on quick cook grains, lentils and other canned pulses will provide a ready supply of simple, nourishing foods. Cold breakfasts, being already cold, save you the disappointment when you finally get around to eating them past noon.

Feeding Your Baby

Throughout the peripartum period a mother constantly, and unknowingly, provides teachings that prepare a baby for the big wide world. When nursing, the nature of breast milk changes over a day, so that at night-time, it is rich in circadian hormones and certain amino acids that help lull a baby to sleep. Breast milk is complex and dynamic — a living fluid that is replete in nutrients and many other things, including microorganisms and biological factors, which nurture a baby's immature immune system.

As a baby's needs change, the components in breast milk shift over time. However, the teachings in breast milk do not flow one way, like a monologue. Breastfeeding is a dialogue between a mother and a baby — an intimate conversation, where a mother imparts what she knows, and a baby, likewise. For instance, when a baby is ill, a mother senses this

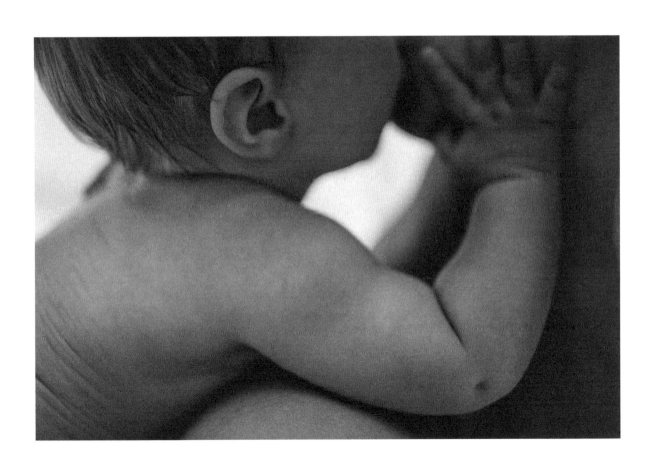

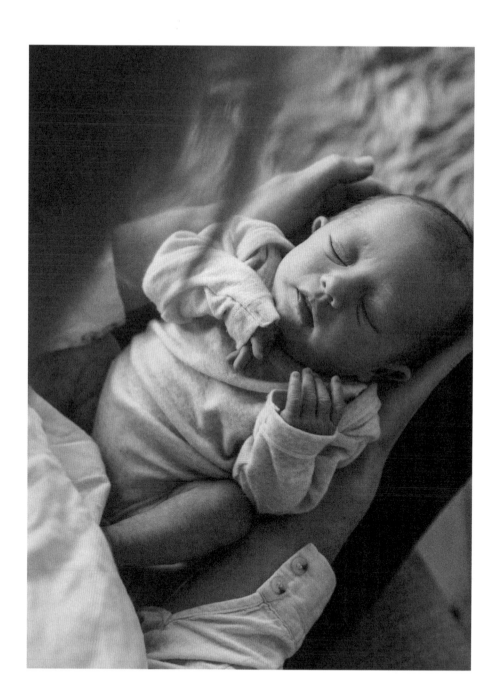

through a change in a baby's saliva and responds by increasing the amount of immunity-boosting compounds in her milk.[158]

Part of what a mother's milk 'knows' is informed by what she eats — her foodways, together with her nutritional reserves and nutrients her body makes, *become* her milk. In effect, breast milk is an embodiment of a mother. It is especially rich in fats that provide a concentrated energy supply to support a baby's rapid growth, as well as the materials needed to build cell membranes, especially those found in fatty brain tissue.

As the fats in breast milk are so important for a baby's growth and development, the total amount of fat in breast milk remains fairly constant, regardless of what is eaten.[159] In other words, fattier breast milk can't be made by eating fattier foods. However, breast milk contains over 200 different fatty acids and the foods that are eaten do affect the proportions of these, including levels of essential omega-3 fats.[160] The amounts of some other nutrients can also vary depending on maternal foodways, including several vitamins, selenium and iodine.[161, 162]

And so, while breast milk is magical, it is not without work, and a mother will need to increase the amount of nourishing foods eaten over the course of a day to avoid becoming (potentially further) depleted. Fortunately, the postpartum season is not layered with the same concerns around food poisoning and avoidances as it is during pregnancy, although there are some considerations around the effects of drinking alcohol, or tea, coffee and other caffeine-containing items, on breast milk (see pages 72, 73).

Getting Started

At birth, a baby is entirely dependent on caregivers, yet will intuitively know how to suckle. A mother, however, does not hold the same instinct. Her body will produce and release milk without thinking, of course. But the practice of feeding a baby, whether by breasts, bottles or both, involves more than producing milk or mixing formula, and must be learnt. This takes time, patience, compassion, but most of all, community.

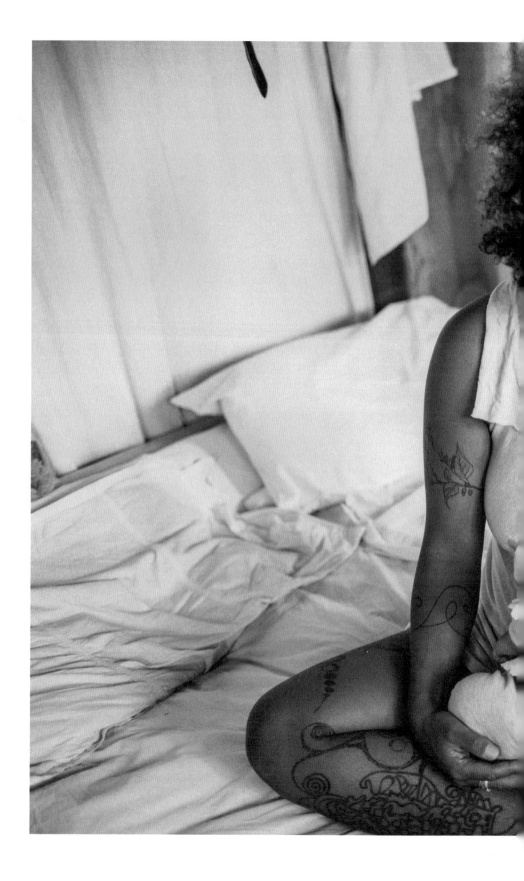

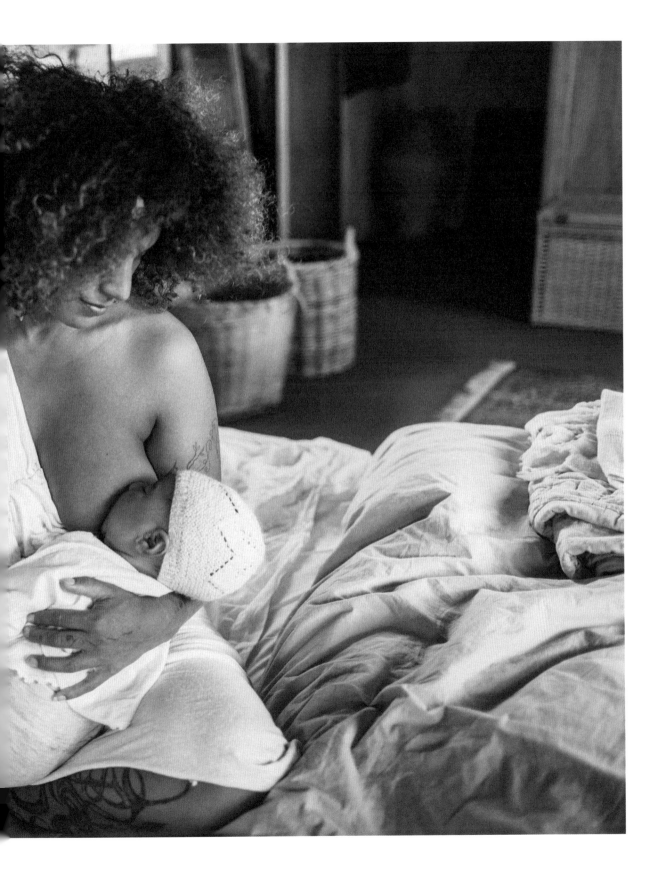

I invite you to let go of any expectations you hold for yourself at this time. Know that transitions may be messy and hazy and splattered with the tears of exhaustion, but that this is simply the way of it — of weaving new connections. Just as our foodways are, feeding your baby is about far more than nutrition. When feeding, your baby can hear your heartbeat and they are reassured by your presence — your touch and smell. Feeding your baby is about connection and it is from closeness that the nourishment and comfort flows.

To establish breastfeeding, ideally your baby will experience skin-to-skin contact and be put on your breast within the first hour of birth. From thereon in, it is advisable to nurse at least 10 to 12 times a day (over 24 hours). Look for early hunger cues including stirring, rooting or hands in mouth. Allow unlimited time at the breast, when actively sucking, and then offer the second breast. If you are unsure, it is a good idea to have a friend who has breastfed or a health professional nearby when nursing the first few times. They can offer reassurance and support on practising good technique, including latch and positioning.

The first milk you produce is rich, fatty and golden and is known as *colostrum*. Colostrum contains many beneficial compounds that support a baby's growth and provide immune protection.[163] You will produce colostrum in very small amounts. After two to five days, your milk will 'come in' and there will be a noticeable difference in the amount, colour and consistency of your milk. Your breasts may feel full, sometimes uncomfortably so. Nurse regularly to minimise engorgement, while you and your baby work together to find a rhythm that works well.

You may notice that breastfeeding increases your appetite. This is your body telling you that she would welcome more nourishment. Similarly, nursing can bring with it an instantaneous, almost unquenchable thirst. It is a good idea to keep a full bottle of water nearby, so that you can grab it when the need to nurse may catch you off guard.

How often and how long a baby will nurse will depend on a few things, including how much milk is available when the breasts are offered,

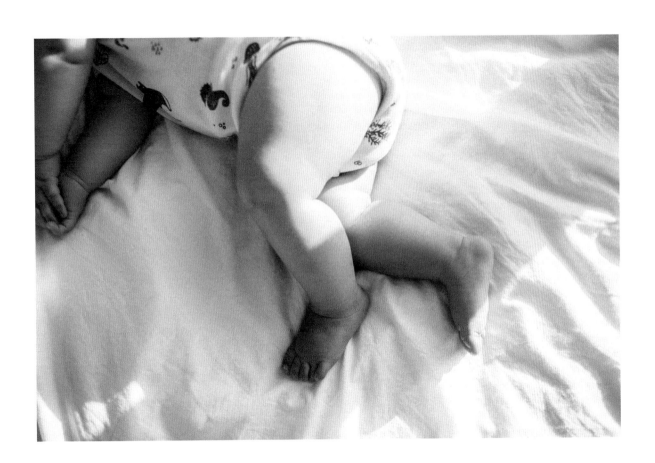

the space in a baby's stomach to hold the milk, and how long it takes for their stomach to empty. Especially in the early days when establishing breastfeeding, you may need to wake your baby to feed, regardless of the time of day. This is because babies can sometimes sleep through hunger cues and emptying the breasts is important to provide a signal to the body to make more milk.

As a general guide, wake your baby to nurse if they have gone two hours since a feed during the day, and four hours at night. In the early weeks, night feeds are important and can contribute a fifth of a baby's daily intake of breast milk. After a month or so, the rhythm of breastfeeding is usually more settled, but continued night feeds are not uncommon.

In your baby's first circle around the sun, there will come many times when they wake for the moon. And in the darkness and stillness of night-time, it may seem like there is only the two of you. Everyone else is tucked away, sound asleep. Or too far away for you to imagine — busy in the daylight — oblivious to the quiet sounds of a hungry baby filling their tummy. In the moment, these times may be shrouded in sleepiness and your body may ache from the punctured sleep and relentless physical demands of early motherhood. It is hard to see in the dark. But long after, you realise that it is these times, like catching the early butterfly kicks and seeing your baby for the first time, that hold the wonder of it all.

Milk Concerns

We may have in our minds an idea of what 'normal' breastfeeding will be like, but we cannot ever know ahead of experiencing it. The nature and rhythm of breastfeeding varies widely and is fluid in response to a baby's needs, which will inevitably change. There may come times when you notice appreciable shifts in number and length of feeds. This is especially common after around three months, when your baby's rate of growth slows. Other changes in feeding practices that may concern you, include your baby being unsettled between or during feeds or appearing to settle 'better'

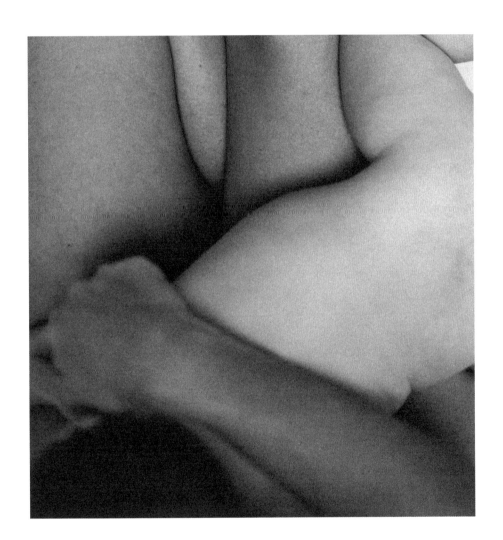

after formula feeds, if offered. You may also notice that your breasts feel softer or empty or your baby's pattern of sucking or swallowing change.

Motherhood can be fraught with worry. While it is understandable that these happenings may concern you, they are generally not helpful indications that there are issues with your feeding practices or milk supply. Instead, it is better to look at the number of wet and soiled nappies, alertness, skin colour, muscle tone, weight gain and growth. If you are worried that your baby is not feeding well, it is important to reach out for help from an experienced friend or family member, local breastfeeding support group or an appropriately trained healthcare professional, such as a breastfeeding counsellor.

It is possible that a woman is unable to produce enough milk, although this is rare. *Primary breastfeeding insufficiency* is the term for when there is not enough glandular breast tissue to sustain breastfeeding and is estimated to affect 5 per cent of mothers. Other factors that may lead to low milk supply include (but are not limited to) retained placental fragments which maintain maternal progesterone levels, and severe illnesses such as extreme postpartum haemorrhage. More common is *secondary breastfeeding insufficiency*, which is the term for when milk is not thoroughly and regularly removed from the breasts, signalling to the body to make less.

Practices and preparations to enhance milk supply

There are ways of adapting nursing practices to signal to the body to produce more milk. Increasing the frequency of nursing day and night and switching sides several times, ensuring the breasts are well drained, can help. Noticing, as well, a baby's nursing technique — are they latching properly or are there factors that may be preventing this, like tongue tie, sleepiness, position or anatomy? Sometimes it's difficult to gauge whether any of these factors are coming into play. If you are worried about your supply or nursing practices, seek help as soon as you can. Remember, nursing is a learnt practice. Before I continue, it is important to emphasise that these practices to promote milk production should be encouraged in

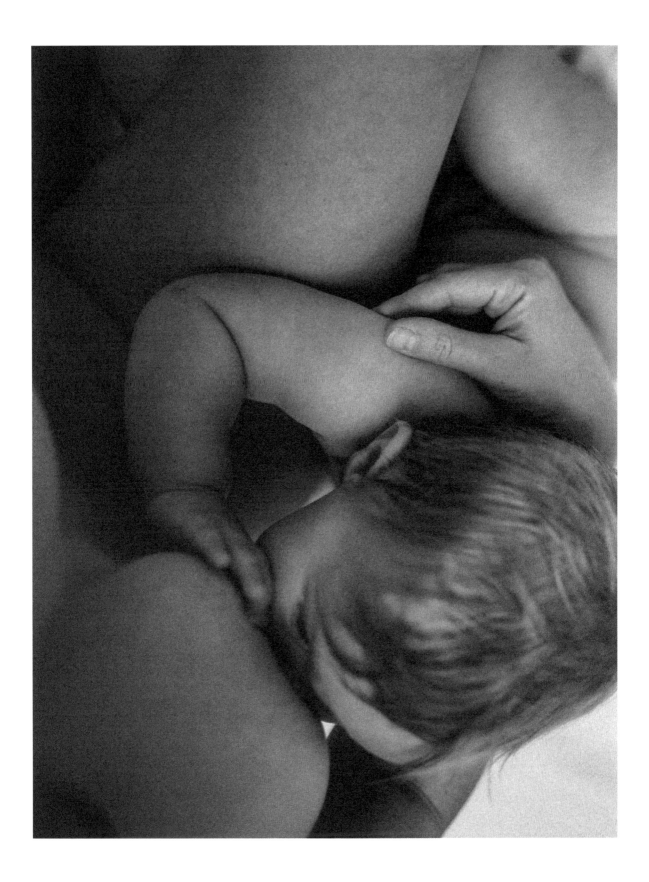

the first instance, as the impact of these will be much more significant than the preparations, I discuss hereafter.

As breast milk is produced partly from foodways, when there are concerns around supply, it makes good sense to look to what a mother is eating. *Galactogogues* are foods, herbs or drugs believed or known to promote breast milk production. Although natural galactogogues are often dismissed by medical practitioners, there is growing evidence, at least for some, of a beneficial effect. If we respect that foods interact with our bodies in many ways we don't fully understand, it is not a stretch to appreciate that some foods may actively promote milk production ahead of others.

There are endless foods and preparations used for their perceived milk-promoting effects — from the traditional quinoa soup enjoyed by Indigenous women in Peru (see Quinoa, Potato and Corn Soup with Sweet Yellow Chilli, page 219), to the dried, crushed earthworms used by some communities in India.[164] There is no room to explore all galactogogues here. Instead, I will briefly discuss fenugreek, as there is some scientific backing for its use, and it is widely available and inexpensive.

FENUGREEK SEEDS

Fenugreek (*Trigonella foenum graecum*) is the most widely studied galactogogue, however, the results of its effects are mixed. Fenugreek stimulates sweat production and since the breasts are made of similar glandular tissue, it may promote milk production this way. The suggested dose of fenugreek is 200 ml thrice daily as a herbal tea or 600 mg thrice daily as a supplement, for one to three weeks.[165] Fenugreek often imparts what has been described as a maple syrup smell, which is nothing to be concerned about. Since fenugreek imbues a delicious earthy flavour to dishes, you will find I use it in a few of my recipes, including Coconut Yoghurt and Lemon Dahl with Sticky Jasmine Rice (page 206).[9]

---

9   Note that sometimes women are dissuaded from eating fenugreek during pregnancy, however, there is no evidence that I am aware of that eating moderate amounts of fenugreek in pregnancy poses any health risk.

Food sensitivities

It is possible, though uncommon, for babies to be sensitive to certain components in breast milk, which originally came from a mother's foodways. [166] Rare cases of allergic reactions to cow's milk protein (not lactose) and fish have been reported. Other signs of food sensitivity may include fussiness and discomfort after feeds, difficulty sleeping, crying, skin irritation, for example eczema, or an upset tummy including sore bottom and/or green stools. Given that these symptoms could be caused by other things, it is important to rule these out before needlessly culling suspected foods.

If you suspect your baby may have a food sensitivity, it is a good idea to keep a diary of what you are eating and the symptoms your baby is experiencing and see if there is a possible connection. To confirm a sensitivity, eliminate the food for several weeks and see if there is any improvement in your baby's symptoms. If symptoms improve, it is important to reintroduce the food to your diet (this is called a challenge) and see if your baby has a reaction. If there is no reaction, then it is unlikely your baby is sensitive to that food. If you would like support with this process, speak with your health professional.

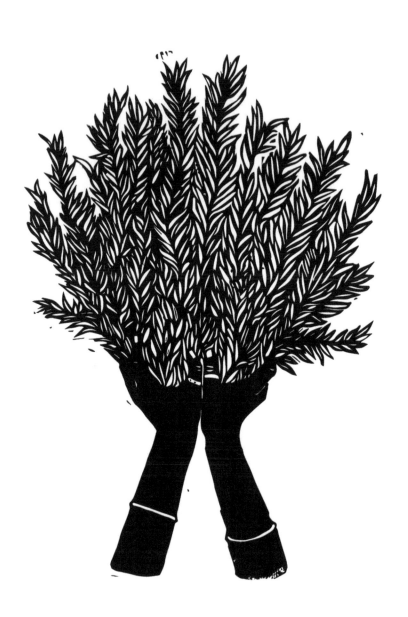

Chapter 7

RECIPES

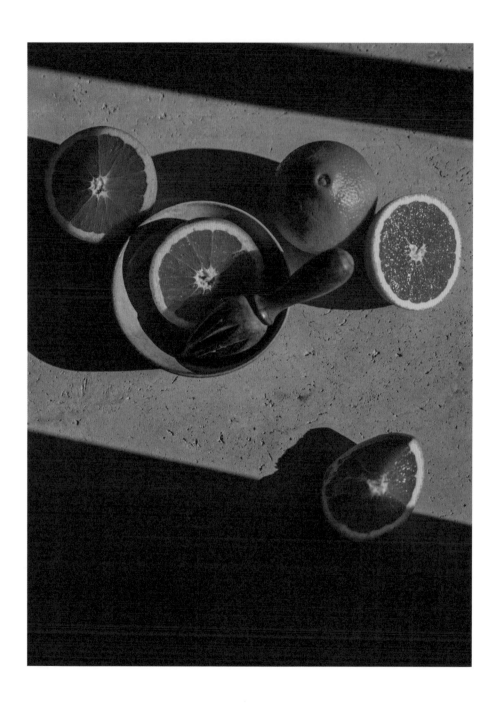

Hereafter you will find some of my favourite seasonal recipes that I turn to time and again. All the dishes are made from plants alone, though it is not my intention in doing so to suggest that eating only plants is the best way of food for people and planet (there is no single best way). Rather, I aim to show how plants can be the greater part of our foodways, without feeling that something is missing. Though on first glance a few dishes seem to take much longer than you might have time for, most are rather hands-off, with a lot of the time taken up with waiting for the stove to work her magic.

Cooking Notes

Measures — Although I have included ingredient volumes (cups) for baked goods, it is better to use weight (grams), as the volume that ingredients can take up can vary the weight considerably — weighing is more accurate. The tablespoons I have used are 20 ml (4 teaspoons). If you are using a smaller 15 ml tablespoon (3 teaspoons), add an extra teaspoon (5 ml) to make up the full amount.

Salt — Where important, I specify fine or coarse salt. Otherwise, you can use whatever salt you prefer.

Stock — I have not specified what sort of stock to use. All the recipes have been tested with vegetable stock, but some would work well with meat or fish stocks.

Flaxseeds/Chia seeds/Eggs — I have used seeds in place of eggs in some recipes. It is possible to use eggs in their place and I have provided directions for doing so. Note that using eggs rather than seeds in baking will give more rise and the crumb of cakes will hold together better.

ZESTY OAT *and* ALMOND LIGHTLY TOASTED MUESLI *with* APRICOTS

Spring/Summer

It is worthwhile making your own toasted muesli at home. You can ensure it contains a trove of good-quality ingredients, which, unlike ready-made products, means that you do not need liberal amounts of added fats and sugars to make up for their missing flavour. Store-bought versions can also sometimes taste a little bitter. This is a sign that the fats in their ingredients have gone rancid and are no longer good for you.

This recipe is simple to pull together from a handful of pantry ingredients. Enjoy this muesli served with fresh, seasonal fruit and a milk of your choosing.

Makes *about 460 g (4 cups)*
Time *30 minutes*

1 orange
285 g (3 cups) rolled oats
50 g (¼ cup) sunflower seeds
1 teaspoon ground cinnamon
2 tablespoons local honey or maple syrup
2 tablespoons extra-virgin olive oil, mild flavour
50 g (½ cup) flaked almonds
125 g (¾ cup) whole dried apricots, sulphite-free, roughly chopped

Preheat the oven to 180°C. Line 2 regular baking trays with parchment paper.

Zest the orange into a large bowl. Add the oats, seeds and cinnamon and set aside.

Juice the orange into a separate bowl or wide-mouth jug. Stir in the honey (or maple syrup) and olive oil. Pour into the bowl with the muesli and mix well.

Spread the muesli out on the tray and toast in the oven for 10 minutes.

Remove the tray from the oven. Stir through the almonds and turn over the muesli ingredients, ready to toast the other side. Return to the oven for a further 5 minutes. Keep your eye on the muesli to avoid burning. Remove and stir through the apricots.

Serve warm or store for up to a week in an airtight container.

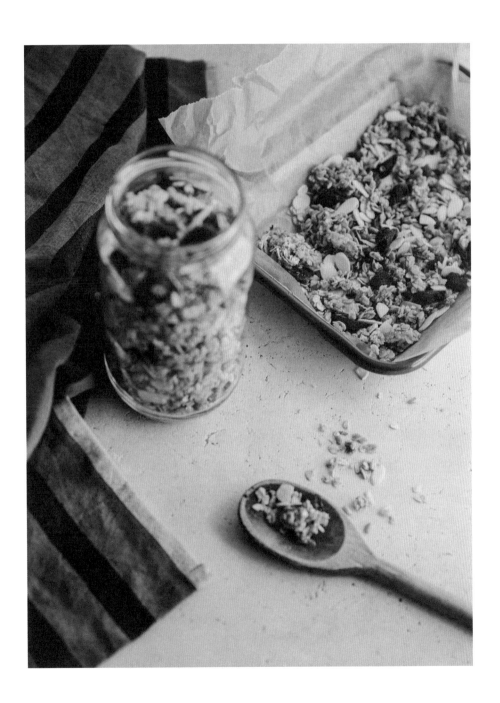

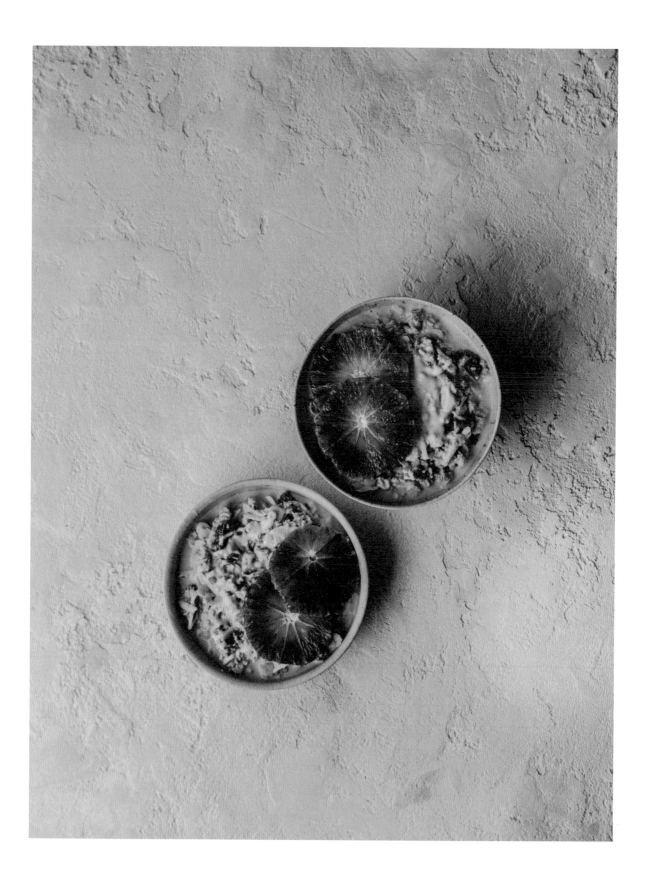

CASHEW YOGHURT
BIRCHER MUESLI

All seasons

With all the haphazard distractions that family life brings, the softened, cool, creamy oats in bircher muesli will wait patiently for you until you're ready. A make-ahead meal your future self will undoubtedly love you for.

Serves *2 generously*
Time *10 minutes, plus refrigerating overnight*

250 g (2 cups) zesty oat and almond muesli (see page 150) or good quality store-bought muesli
375 ml (1½ cups) milk of your choice
1 eating apple, cored and grated with peel
2 tablespoons toasted cashew yoghurt (see page 253) or unsweetened Greek yoghurt
seasonal fruit to top

Place the muesli in a large bowl and pour over the milk. Stir to combine, then cover with a tea towel or plate and refrigerate overnight.

In the morning the muesli should have soaked up most, if not all of the milk. Grate in the apple and a spoonful of the yoghurt. Mix well then spoon the bircher evenly into two bowls. Top each bowl with a dollop of cashew yoghurt and some seasonal fruit.

BERRY, COCONUT
and OAT THICKIE

Spring/Summer/Autumn

I used to work for a smoothie company in London and one of their products was the inspiration for this recipe. It was called a 'Raspberry Thickie' and was my favourite product. I would enjoy a thickie every morning for second breakfast, until I came to work one day, and just like that, it had been discontinued. Perhaps I was a lone fan, but don't let that put you off my version. This is tangy and filling and something you can smugly prepare the night before, ready for those hazy motherhood mornings. If you don't have coconut yoghurt, try a thick and tart Greek yoghurt instead.

Serves *2*
Time *5 minutes*

260 g (1 cup) coconut yoghurt, unsweetened
250 g (2 cup) mixed berries, e.g. raspberries, blueberries
1 Granny Smith apple, peeled, cored and chopped
2 handfuls of rolled oats
local honey or maple syrup to taste

Blend all the ingredients in a food processor to get a thick and pulpy consistency. Serve in a bowl with a spoon, or drink from a glass.

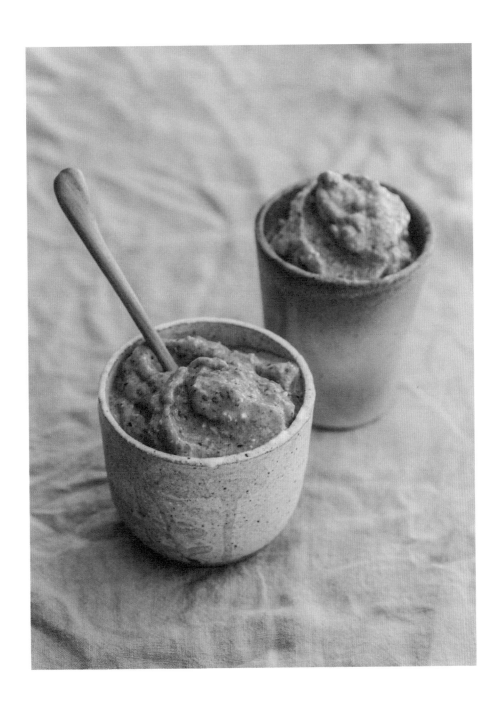

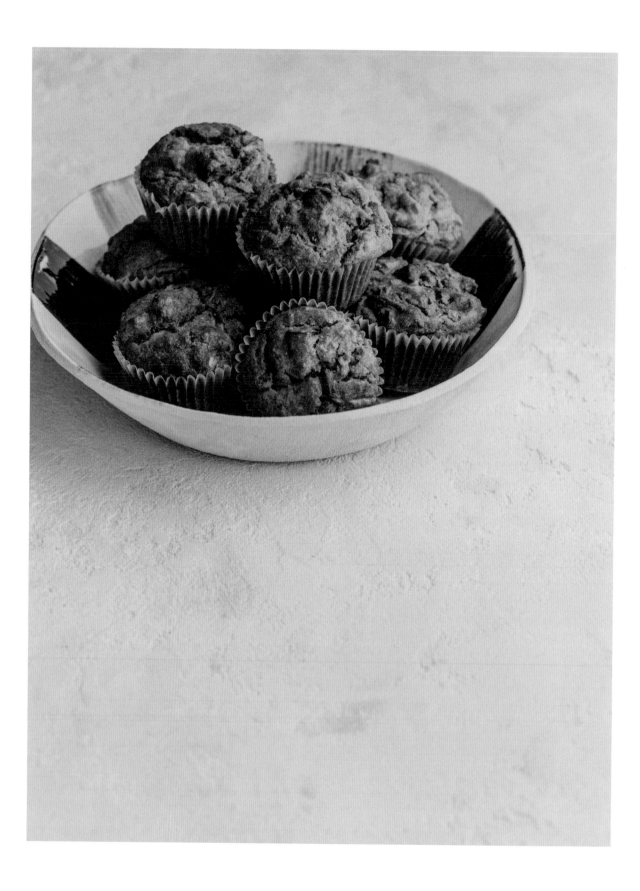

WHOLE WHEAT PORRIDGE MUFFINS *with* APPLES *and* DATES

All seasons

Blessed is the day when we win in making just the right amount of porridge for our family — when there is not too much nor too little, and everyone around the table can start the day well. Far more often than not, this porridge-making heaven remains elusive to us. And while we can add extra nuts, fruit and milk to our bowls to eke out a shortfall, the question of what to do with the surplus usually has us scratching our heads, even after our coffee has kicked in. Normally, we will hold onto leftovers and add these to the next day's porridge pot, but it is handy to have a recipe that makes good use of extras.

I must confess, I did not invent porridge muffins, but other recipes I tried were somewhat disappointing. I hope these are not. I have found that the trick to a good muffin from this recipe is stirring through the porridge well — a pocket of rubbery porridge is as unfortunate as it sounds. If your porridge is cold when you come to make these, it can be a good idea to set it on the stove to briefly warm it through and soften it up again.

Makes *9–12 muffins*
Time *30 minutes*

185 ml (¾ cup) milk of your choice
120 g (1 cup) pitted dried dates, roughly chopped
150 g (1 cup) whole wheat flour
2 tablespoons rapadura sugar
1 tablespoon ground flaxseeds (linseeds) or 1 egg, beaten (see note)
1½ teaspoons baking powder, aluminium-free
1 teaspoon ground cinnamon
½ teaspoon bicarbonate of soda
225 g (1 cup) porridge
145 ml (½ cup + 1 tablespoon) extra-virgin olive oil, mild flavour
2 eating apples, peeled and grated

For the cinnamon sugar
1 teaspoon rapadura sugar
¼ teaspoon ground cinnamon

Preheat the oven to 180°C. Line a 12-cup muffin tin with paper cases.

Warm the milk in a small saucepan over a low–medium heat and immediately remove from the heat just before it reaches a boil. Add the dates and set aside to soften, about 10 minutes.

Meanwhile, whisk the flour, sugar, flaxseeds, baking powder, cinnamon and bicarbonate of soda together in a large mixing bowl.

Combine the date-milk mixture with the dry ingredients along with the porridge, olive oil and apple. Stir until the porridge is well mixed and no flour is visible then spoon the batter into the paper cases.

Make the cinnamon sugar by stirring the sugar and cinnamon together in a small bowl, then sprinkle evenly over the muffin tops.

Bake the muffins until cooked through and a skewer inserted into the centre comes out clean, about 30 minutes. Transfer to a cooling rack and cool before eating.

NOTE
If using an egg in place of flaxseeds, add this with the wet ingredients (the porridge, olive oil and apple).

TERIYAKI TOFU *and* GREEN BEAN BOWL *with* QUICK PICKLED CUCUMBER

Spring / Summer / Autumn

Gluten-free (use tamari)

This make-ahead recipe is just as good for dinner as it is for breakfast. Tofu is best left overnight to soak up the flavour of the marinade. The pickled cucumber is sharp and fresh and will wake you up, as all good breakfasts should.

Serves *4*
Time *30 minutes (split the night before and at breakfast)*

80 ml (⅓ cup) tamari or soy sauce
80 ml (⅓ cup) local honey or maple syrup
2 tablespoons rice wine vinegar
1 tablespoon cornflour
4 cloves garlic, minced
a knob of ginger, minced
375 g firm tofu, pressed and cubed (see notes)
toasted sesame oil
250 g green beans, topped and chopped
300 g (1½ cups) long-grain rice, cooked ahead

For the pickled cucumber
250 ml (1 cup) vinegar, e.g. white, cider or rice wine vinegar
250 ml (1 cup) water
1 tablespoon rapadura sugar (optional)
4 Lebanese cucumbers, thickly sliced on the diagonal

The night before, whisk the tamari (or soy sauce), honey (or maple syrup), vinegar, cornflour, garlic and ginger together until well combined. Pour into a small saucepan and heat gently for a minute or two, stirring regularly, until bubbles form at the edges. Remove from the heat and continue stirring until the marinade thickens.

Pour into a bowl or glass container and add the tofu. Cover with a plate or lid and shake the tofu so it is well coated in the marinade. Refrigerate overnight.

For the cucumber, take a sterilised jar (see notes) and combine the vinegar, water and sugar and stir well. Add the cucumbers and refrigerate overnight.

In the morning, warm a generous splash of sesame oil in a large frying pan or wok over a medium–high heat. Add the tofu and green beans and stir-fry until they are charred and cooked through on all sides, about 6–8 minutes.

Serve with the cooked rice and cucumbers on the side.

NOTES

To remove excess water from tofu for better flavour and texture, you can either use a tofu press or create a makeshift version. To do so, take a plate and place on it a clean dry tea towel folded in half, with half the towel hanging to the side. Rest the tofu in the centre of the towel on the plate, then bring over the tea towel to cover it. Place another plate on top of the covered tofu and something heavy on top of the plate to press out any liquid. I have a heavy teapot that does this job nicely, but a heavy bowl or similar would work just as well. Leave the tofu for at least 30 minutes, after which, the tea towel will be damp.

To sterilise a jar, first preheat the oven to 160°C. Wash the jar and lid in hot, soapy water. While they are still wet, stand them upside down on a roasting tray and transfer to the oven. Heat for 15 minutes then carefully remove the jar and lid and place on a tea towel ready to fill.

HAZELNUT, WHOLE WHEAT *and* BUTTERMILK PANCAKES *with* APPLE

All seasons

As pancakes need a little more attention than the simpler breakfasts we eat on weekdays, they are reserved as a weekend ritual in our home. These pancakes will fill your kitchen with the sweet smell of toasted hazelnut. I have used ready-ground hazelnuts in this recipe, but if you can, it is best to make your own by blitzing them from whole nuts in a food processor. Without a doubt, they will taste better.

Makes *about 12 pancakes*
Time *40 minutes*

310 ml (1¼ cups) milk of your choice
2 teaspoons lemon juice or apple cider vinegar
185 g (1¼ cups) whole wheat flour
70 g (⅓ cup) rapadura sugar
55 g (½ cup) ground hazelnuts
1 tablespoon chia seeds or 1 egg, beaten (see note)
½ teaspoon bicarbonate of soda
a pinch of fine salt
60 ml (¼ cup) extra-virgin coconut oil, melted and cooled, plus extra for frying
1 eating apple, cored and finely sliced
ground cinnamon to serve

Whisk the milk and lemon juice (or vinegar) together in a jug. Set aside until the milk turns clumpy like buttermilk, about 5 minutes.

Mix the flour, sugar, ground hazelnuts, chia seeds, bicarbonate of soda and salt in a large bowl. Pour in the buttermilk mixture and coconut oil and stir the batter until no flour is visible, but do not overmix. Leave the batter to stand and thicken, about 10 minutes (or overnight in fridge).

Preheat the oven to keep the pancakes warm while you fry the full batch.

While the batter thickens, warm a large frying pan over a medium heat, ensuring the pan is not so hot that the oil will smoke. Spare a couple of minutes to ensure the oil has warmed through. When you are ready to begin frying, add a couple of teaspoons of coconut oil for each pancake. Allow around 1 heaped tablespoon of batter per pancake and gently coax the batter into a circle with the back of the spoon. Lightly press 2 or 3 apple slices into the batter. When the pancake bubbles and browns a little at the edges, after a minute or so, flip it over and fry the other side. If your pan is large enough, you can fry 3 or 4 pancakes at the same time.

Once cooked, transfer the pancakes to an ovenproof dish and place in the warm oven. Continue making pancakes until the batter is used up. In between batches, clear any scattered bits of batter, so they do not burn in the pan.

Serve warm with a good sprinkle of ground cinnamon.

> NOTE
> *If using an egg in place of chia seeds, add this with the wet ingredients (the buttermilk mixture and coconut oil).*

MARMALADE LOAF *with* WALNUTS

All seasons

The marmalade in this cake joyously bubbles and pops when retrieved from its hot oven home. This is best enjoyed while still warm, with a hot cup of tea.

Makes *1 loaf*
Time *50 minutes*

2 tablespoons ground flaxseeds (linseeds) or 2 eggs, beaten
150 g (1 cup) whole wheat flour
120 g (1 cup) rye flour
90 g (⅔ cup) rapadura sugar
60 g (½ cup) walnuts, roughly chopped
50 g (½ cup) rolled oats
85 g (½ cup) sultanas
2 teaspoons baking powder, aluminium-free
1 teaspoon ground cinnamon
½ teaspoon bicarbonate of soda
125 ml (½ cup) extra-virgin olive oil (mild flavour)
310 ml (1¼ cups) milk of your choice
2 tablespoons orange marmalade with peel

Preheat the oven to 180°C. Grease and line a (22 cm x 11 cm) loaf pan.

Whisk the flaxseeds with 100 ml water. Leave to thicken, about 5 minutes. If using egg, add to the wet ingredients (the olive oil and milk).

Combine the flours, sugar, walnuts, oats, sultanas, baking powder, cinnamon and bicarbonate of soda in a large bowl and mix well. In a jug, whisk the olive oil and milk (and eggs, if using), then pour into the bowl of dry ingredients, along with 1 tablespoon of the marmalade, and gently stir to combine until no flour is visible.

Pour the batter into the loaf pan and tap its base on the kitchen bench a couple of times to remove any air pockets and even out the mixture. Spoon the second tablespoon of marmalade on top of the mixture, spreading it evenly with the back of the spoon.

Bake until golden and bubbly on top, and a skewer inserted in the middle comes out clean, about 40 minutes. Leave in the pan for a few minutes so it is cool enough to handle and transfer to a cooling rack.

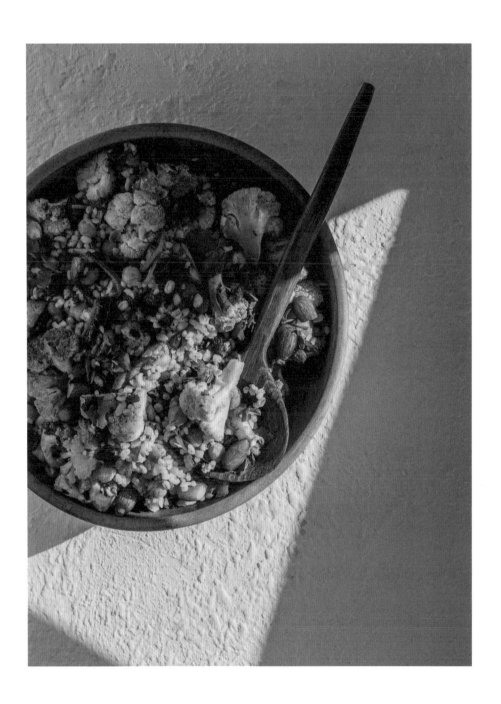

ROAST CAULIFLOWER, CHICKPEA *and* BULGUR SALAD *with* RAS EL HANOUT

Spring / Autumn / Winter
Gluten-free

Ras el hanout is a North African spice blend that is customarily used as a rub or stirred through grains or in a tagine. In Arabic, ras el hanout translates to 'head of the shop' — meaning a mix of the very best spices a merchant has to offer. There is no definitive recipe for ras el hanout, but it will often include cardamom, cassia, mace, clove, cumin, chilli and dried rose petals. It is usually full of flavour but is not necessarily 'hot' spicy.

This salad is one of my favourites, if not my number one recipe in this book. It is really easy to prepare but packed with flavour, and quite versatile — you could try other dried fruit such as dates and apricots, and couscous or brown rice would work in place of bulgur.

Serves *4*
Time *45 minutes*

1 head of a good size cauliflower
1 red onion, quartered and thinly sliced
ras el hanout
extra-virgin olive oil
salt
400 g (2 cups or 2 x 400-g cans) cooked chickpeas, rinsed and drained
80 g (½ cup) almonds, roughly chopped
175 g (1 cup) bulgur
120 g (⅔ cup) raisins or sultanas
a handful of fresh parsley, finely chopped

Preheat the oven to 200°C.

Chop the cauliflower into small florets and dice the core. Roughly chop and set aside any leaves. Spread out the cauliflower and red onion in a roasting dish, sprinkle over a good amount (e.g. a couple of tablespoons) of ras el hanout, drizzle well with olive oil and sprinkle over a good pinch of salt. Toss to coat.

Roast until cooked through and brown in places, about 40 minutes. Halfway through, add the chickpeas, almonds and another drizzle of olive oil. A few minutes before the cauliflower is done, add the cauliflower leaves with another little drizzle of olive oil.

Meanwhile, in a medium saucepan bring 625 ml (2½ cups) water to the boil. Add bulgur, cover and simmer until cooked through and the water is absorbed, about 15–20 minutes.

Combine the bulgur with the roast cauliflower mix and stir through the raisins (or sultanas) and parsley. Enjoy hot or cold.

PUMPKIN FARROTTO *with* CRISPY SHREDDED KALE *and* SAGE

Autumn / Winter

Farrotto is a traditional Tuscan risotto made with farro rather than rice. Although farro is sometimes used as a general term for spelt, emmer and einkorn, each are actually different species of wheat — *farro grande* (spelt), *farro medio* (emmer) and *farro piccolo* (einkorn). Farro without any descriptor of size (big, medium, small) usually refers to medio/medium — emmer wheat. The word emmer is derived from *'Em ha'Hitah'*, which in Hebrew means 'mother wheat', stemming from its use since the very advent of farming. Emmer has a malty flavour that is so delicious with the pumpkin, nutmeg and sage, that it is worth tracking some down. If you don't have emmer, then pearl barley would be a good substitute, or at a push, arborio rice would also be fine and will cook far quicker.

Serves *4*
Time *1 hour 10 minutes*

extra-virgin olive oil
1 brown onion, diced
4 cloves garlic, minced
300 g (1 cup) pearled farro, unwashed
1 whole nutmeg
125 ml (½ cup) dry white wine (see note)
400 g (2⅔ cups) pumpkin, peeled, deseeded and cubed
1¼ litres (5 cups) stock, kept warm in a separate saucepan
2 large handfuls of Tuscan kale (cavolo nero)
a handful of sage leaves, large ones halved lengthways down the stem

Warm a generous splash of olive oil in a large saucepan over a medium heat. Sauté the onion and garlic, stirring regularly, until the onion is soft and translucent, about 10 minutes. Add the farro and a good grating of nutmeg, then stir and toast, adding extra oil if needed so that every grain is coated.

When the farro smells nutty, after about 2 minutes, add the wine and let it simmer until it has all absorbed. Add the pumpkin and enough stock to bathe the

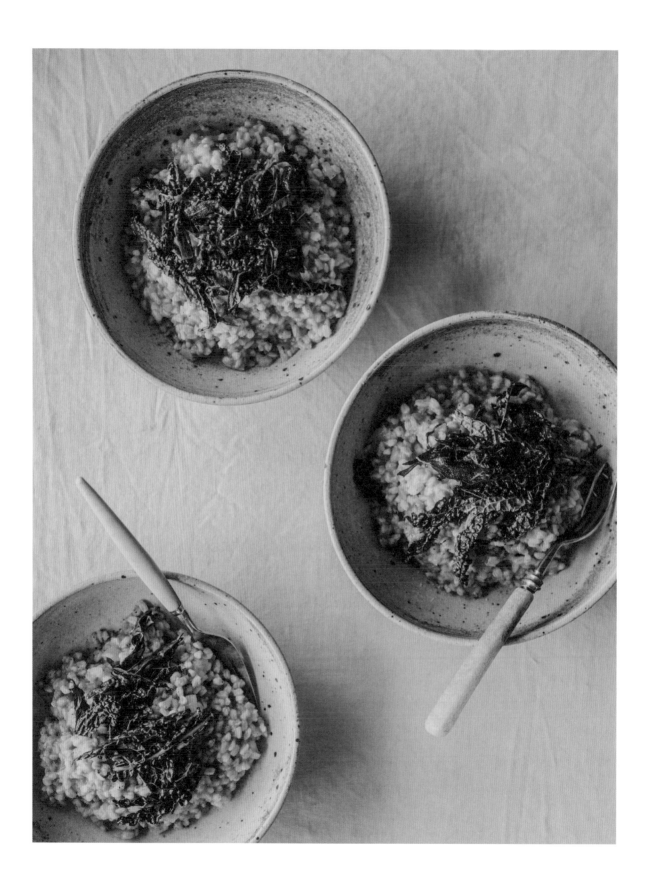

ingredients. Simmer uncovered. As the stock reduces, top up with more until the pumpkin is soft, the farro cooked through and the stock has been used up, about 1 hour. By this time, if the pumpkin hasn't relaxed and softened to create a thick sauce, help it along and mash it into the farrotto with the back of a spatula or a fork.

When the farrotto is nearly ready, shred the kale by folding each leaf in half and then slicing into long thin strips. Remove and compost the tough stems. Warm a generous splash of olive oil in a large frying pan over a medium heat. Add the kale and sage and fry until crispy, about 5 minutes. Top the farrotto with the shredded leaves.

NOTE

When cooking with alcohol, the amount the alcohol will reduce by depends on how long the dish is cooked for. A long-simmered dish like this farrotto will retain around 5 per cent of the alcohol initially added — meaning that a serving will contain a negligible amount (even though the wine adds significantly to its flavour).[167] *In dishes that are cooked briefly, the alcohol remaining can range from 10–50 per cent. If you would prefer not to use wine or have none to hand, simply make up the difference with extra stock.*

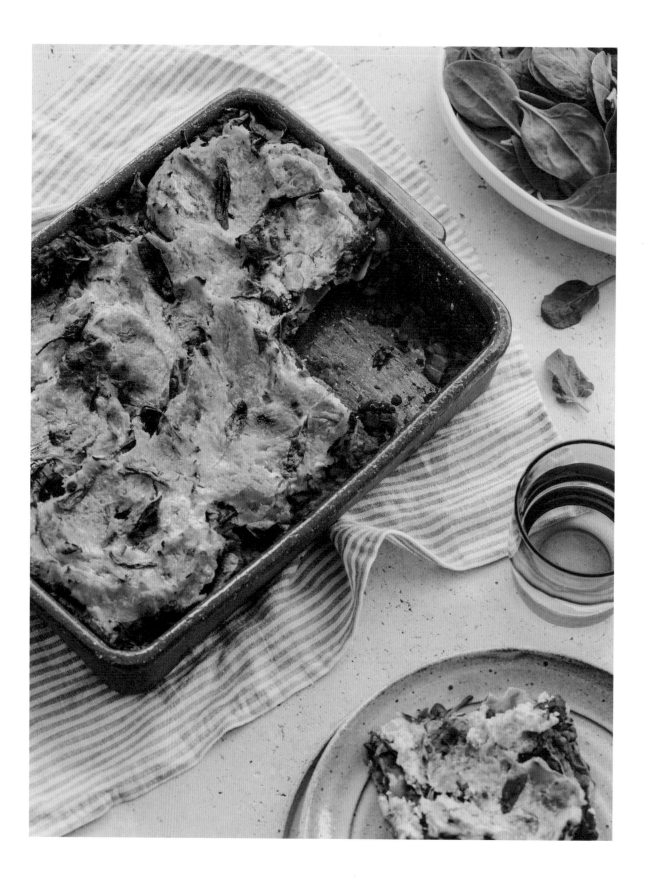

SQUASH, SAGE *and* BABY SPINACH LASAGNE *with* TRIPLE TOMATO LENTILS

Summer/Autumn

This recipe makes a wholesome, hearty lasagne — the kind with lots of layers of colourful goodness that will satisfy even the hungriest of tummies. It is the sort of dish I'd make on a weekend when we have friends coming over for dinner with their children. The creamy squash goes together so well with the rich triple tomato lentils. If you really want to go to town or need to feed a crowd, you could add in some extra layers of thinly sliced zucchini (courgette) or sliced, cooked eggplant (aubergine). Serve with some simple salad leaves dressed lightly with balsamic vinegar or maple-mustard dressing (page 201).

Serves *6–8*
Time *1 hour 30 minutes*

1 large (about 1.5–1.8 kg) butternut squash, peeled, deseeded and cubed
extra-virgin olive oil
salt
1 brown onion, diced
4 cloves garlic, minced
1 teaspoon ground cinnamon
2 teaspoons ground cumin
500 ml (2 cups) passata
400 g (2 cups or 2 x 400 g cans, rinsed and drained) cooked brown lentils
250 g (1 cup) tomato paste
40 g (1 cup) sun-dried tomatoes, chopped
Worcestershire sauce, tamari or soy sauce
1 quantity cultured cashew cream (see page 257) or 230 g (1 cup) ricotta cheese
a handful of fresh sage leaves, stems removed and finely chopped, plus extra for
    garnish
1 whole nutmeg
dried lasagne sheets
2 handfuls of baby spinach leaves

Preheat the oven to 200°C.

Spread out the squash on a roasting tray, drizzle well with olive oil and a good pinch of salt. Toss well to coat. Roast in the oven until cooked through, soft and just starting to brown, about 50 minutes. Toss halfway through.

Meanwhile prepare the tomato lentils. Warm a generous splash of olive oil in a large saucepan over a medium heat. Sauté the onion and garlic, stirring regularly, until the onion is soft and translucent, about 10 minutes. Add the cinnamon and cumin and cook for a few minutes until fragrant, then add the passata, lentils, tomato paste, sun-dried tomatoes and a good splash of Worcestershire sauce (or tamari or soy sauce). Simmer gently, uncovered, to reduce the sauce and combine the flavours, until the squash is ready.

Remove the squash from the oven (keep the oven on) and mash well with the back of a fork or potato masher. Mash through the cashew cream (or ricotta), sage and a good amount of freshly grated nutmeg.

Prepare the lasagne by layering half the tomato lentils into a large ovenproof dish about 30 cm x 24 cm. Cover with a layer of lasagne sheets, then half the squash, and a handful of spinach leaves. Cover with another layer of lasagne sheets, the remaining tomato lentils, a handful of spinach, a final layer of lasagne sheets, and then the remaining squash. Garnish with extra sage leaves and drizzle with a little olive oil.

Return to the oven and cook until the pasta cuts easily with a knife, about 30 minutes.

Leave to cool for 10 minutes before serving.

SPELT BERRY, SUNFLOWER SEED, APRICOT *and* APPLE PILAF *with* CARAWAY

All seasons

Spelt berries are my favourite grain. They are sweet and nutty and, cooked well, are ever so slightly chewy — perfect in grain-based salads like this one. Before the industrialisation of farming, spelt was preferred over wheat and eaten more widely. However, unlike wheat, spelt has a tough outer husk that needs removing before it can be milled into flour and it typically yields lower amounts — factors that count against it in a system that favours efficiency and productivity. It is for reasons like these that large parts of the world have been streamlined into eating just a handful of staple grains (namely wheat, rice and maize/corn) rather than enjoying biodiverse foodways. Fortunately, there is a resurgence of interest in other grains like spelt, and they are now easier to get hold of, though there is still a long way to go. If you cannot find spelt you could try barley or a long-grain brown rice instead.

Serves *2 as a main, 4 as a side*
Time *1 hour 15 minutes*

extra-virgin olive oil
1 red onion, diced
1 stalk celery, diced
2 cloves garlic, minced
200 g (1 cup) spelt berries, preferably soaked overnight
½ teaspoon caraway seeds
1 bay leaf
a pinch of fine salt
ground black pepper
1 large carrot, grated
1 large apple, cored and diced
75 g (½ cup) sunflower seeds
45 g (¼ cup) dried apricots, sulphite-free, roughly chopped
2 large handfuls of rocket (arugula), roughly chopped

Warm a generous splash of olive oil in a large saucepan over a medium heat. Sauté the onion, celery and garlic, stirring regularly, until the onion is soft and translucent, about 10 minutes. Add the spelt berries and caraway seeds and toast for a few minutes until fragrant.

Pour in 625 ml (2½ cups) just-boiled water and the bay leaf, and season with salt and black pepper.

Bring to a boil then reduce the heat to a simmer. Cover and cook until the spelt has started to soften, about 20 minutes. Add the carrot and apple to the pan and stir through. If the pilaf is looking dry, add a dash of water. Cover and cook until the spelt is cooked through, about 20 minutes.

When the pilaf is almost ready, dry toast the sunflower seeds in a frying pan until they smell sweet, about 2–3 minutes. When the pilaf is cooked, remove the bay leaf and stir through the toasted seeds, apricots and rocket.

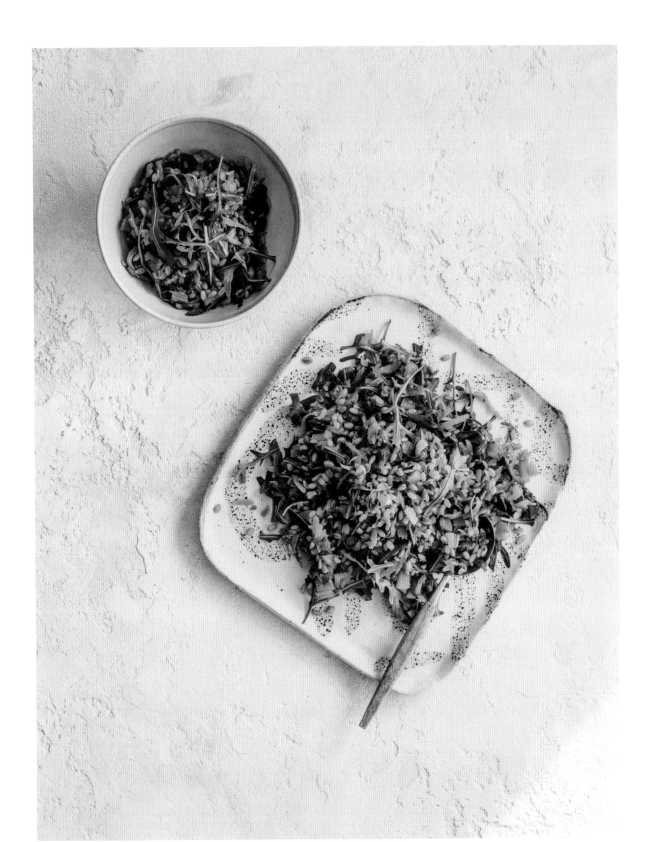

CARAMELISED FENNEL *and*
SUN-DRIED TOMATO PASTA
with CANNELLINI BEANS

Spring/Autumn/Winter

It is not often that I have the time, energy or ingredients to prepare a dish fully from scratch. Finding balance with my home cooking in the bigger picture of my life as a mother involves a little give and take. Here, for example, I am happy to leave the fennel and onions to caramelise a while, so that I can make time for other things that call my attention. I could very well cook the beans from dry, prepare a fresh tomato sauce and make my own pasta, and the meal would taste all the better for it, but using some ready-made options is a compromise I'm happy to make. You can't scrimp on caramelising — this is a practice that is worth doing properly for the flavour, but it simply cannot be hurried. And, in my opinion, nor should it. If all the work is taken out of cooking, the connection is lost.

Serves *4*
Time *1 hour*

extra-virgin olive oil
1 red onion, diced
1 fennel bulb, diced and fronds roughly chopped
1 tablespoon apple cider vinegar
1 tablespoon rapadura sugar or local honey
salt
ground black pepper
4 cloves garlic, minced
1 teaspoon sweet paprika
500 ml (2 cups) passata
200 g (1 cup) cooked or 1 x 400-g can cannellini beans, rinsed and drained
40 g (¼ cup) sun-dried tomato strips, roughly chopped
a small handful fresh oregano leaves, picked from stems, plus extra to serve
500 g (5 cups) dried pasta of your choice

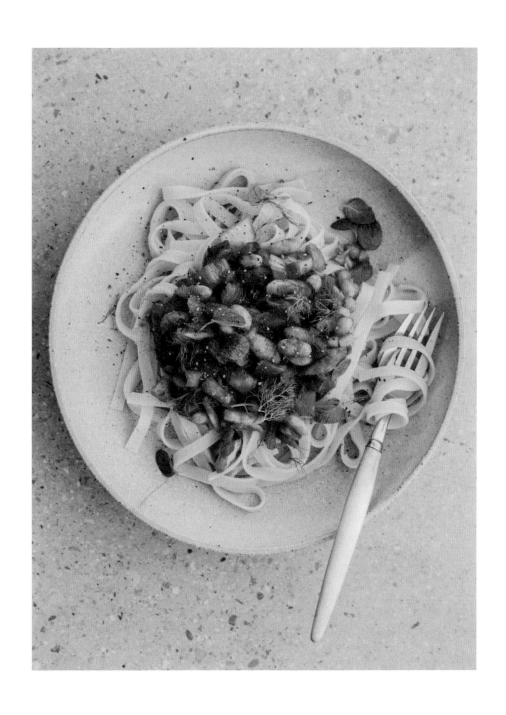

Warm a generous splash of olive oil in a large frying pan over a medium heat. Add the onion, fennel, vinegar, sugar (or honey) and season with salt and pepper. Stir well. Cook over a low–medium heat, stirring occasionally, until the fennel and onion have caramelised, about 30–40 minutes. Add the garlic and paprika and cook for a few minutes more. Follow with the passata, beans, sun-dried tomatoes and oregano. Cook for a couple of minutes over a low heat to warm through.

Prepare the pasta according to packet instructions in salted water. When ready, drain the pasta but catch the cooking water in a jug or bowl. Add 60–125 ml (¼–½ cup) of pasta water to the beans to loosen the sauce.

Serve scattered with fresh oregano and fennel fronds, and ground black pepper.

BLACK BEAN *and* WALNUT BURGERS *with* TOMATO KASUNDI

Spring / Summer / Autumn
Gluten-free (use gluten-free breadcrumbs)

Kasundi is a traditional Bengali chutney made with fermented mustard. Known as 'the queen of the pickles', the preparation of kasundi is steeped in fascinating rules and rituals, which are interesting to read about if you get the chance. Preparation of kasundi was originally rooted in the seasonal availability of mustard and coincided with the first month of the Bengali calendar. After harvesting, women worked in groups and sang songs as they washed the mustard seeds in rivers and ponds.

Over time, as lives and perspectives have shifted, these customs have softened, and some have been lost altogether. The nature of kasundi has changed as well. Traditional kasundi is golden and punchy — very different to modern versions, which are not as pungent and often contain sweet vegetables like tomatoes and eggplant (aubergine). While different, these modern recipes do offer a great entry point to this delicious condiment, which can also be used as a marinade or base for curries.

Makes *8–10 burgers and 550 g (2¼ cups) kasundi*
Time *1 hour 15 minutes*

For the kasundi
extra-virgin olive oil
6 cloves garlic, minced
a knob of fresh ginger, minced
a handful of curry leaves, stalks removed and finely chopped
1 tablespoon yellow mustard seeds
1 tablespoon cumin seeds
1 teaspoon fenugreek seeds
8 plum tomatoes (or similar), skinned (see notes) and roughly chopped
125 ml (½ cup) apple cider vinegar
50 g (¼ cup) rapadura sugar
1 bay leaf
a good pinch of salt

For the burgers

extra-virgin olive oil

1 brown onion, diced

60 g (½ cup) walnuts, preferably soaked overnight, if not, at least 20 minutes

4 cloves garlic

2 teaspoons cumin seeds

1 teaspoon sweet paprika

a pinch of salt

ground black pepper

1 zucchini, grated

1 carrot, grated

400 g (2 cups) cooked black beans or 2 x 400-g cans, rinsed and drained

60 g (1 cup) fresh breadcrumbs (from day-old bread)

a handful of fresh parsley, finely chopped

2 tablespoons ground flaxseeds (linseeds)

Worcestershire or soy sauce

burger buns, salad and homemade chips to serve

To make the kasundi

Warm a generous splash of olive oil in a large saucepan over a medium heat. Sauté the garlic, ginger and curry leaves, stirring regularly until fragrant, about 5 minutes. Add the mustard, cumin and fenugreek seeds to the pan and toast for a couple of minutes. Add the tomatoes, vinegar, sugar, bay leaf and salt, and simmer uncovered for 1 hour. Stir occasionally to prevent burning and remove the bay leaf before serving.

To make the burgers

Warm a generous splash of olive oil in a large frying pan over a medium heat. Sauté the onion, stirring regularly, and cook until soft and translucent, about 10 minutes.

Meanwhile, use a food processor, to mince the walnuts, garlic, cumin, paprika, salt and pepper. Add the walnut mince into the pan with the softened onions, and toast for a couple of minutes. Pour in extra olive oil if the pan is too dry.

Add the grated zucchini and carrot, and black beans and cook until the juices have started to come out of the zucchini, about 5 minutes. Remove the pan from the heat and use a potato masher to briefly mash most of the beans. Empty the mixture into a large bowl and stir through the breadcrumbs, parsley, flaxseeds and a good splash of Worcestershire or soy sauce, until well combined.

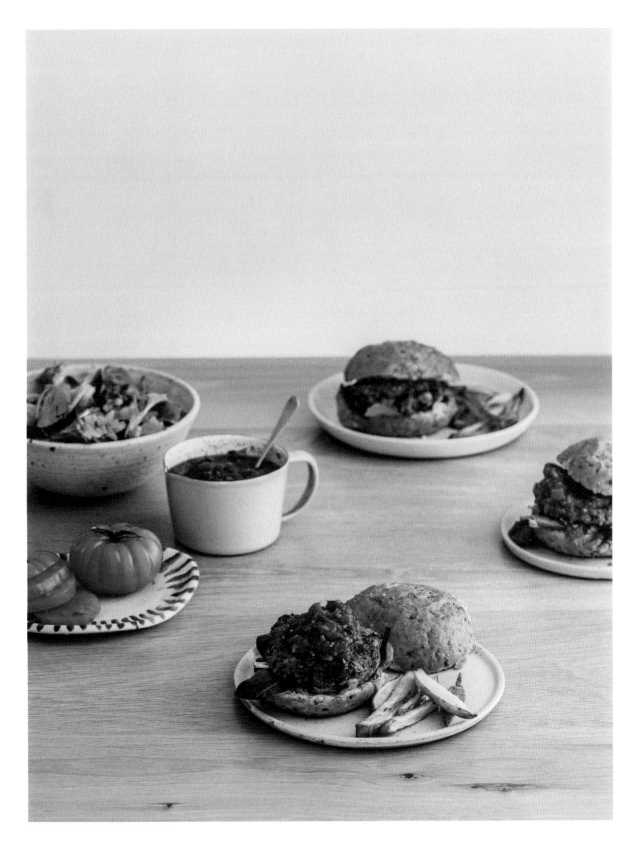

Cover the base of a large frying pan with a thin layer of olive oil and warm over a medium heat. Grab a handful of the burger mix and shape it into a palm-size burger. Carefully place the burger in the frying pan and sear until brown, a few minutes on each side. If your pan is large enough, you can cook several burgers at once. Transfer to a plate while you finish frying the full batch.

To serve, spread the kasundi generously over one half of a burger bun and top with a burger and salad. Try a dollop of kasundi on the side to dip your chips into.

NOTES

To skin tomatoes, use a small knife to score a cross on the bottom of each. Place the tomatoes into a large bowl and cover with just-boiled water. Leave to stand until the skins start to roll back on their own, about 30 seconds. Drain the water and continue to peel away the skin from the tomato.

As a general rule, traditional chutneys are best stored for 4–10 weeks before using and best eaten within one to two years. This kasundi recipe does not have as much vinegar as a chutney usually would as the tomatoes are already acidic, and it can be eaten straight after cooking, but may not store as long. I would recommend keeping the kasundi in a clean, sealed container in the refrigerator and using within a month. It will taste even better after a couple of weeks of storage.

TAMARIND CHICKPEAS *and* COCONUT YOGHURT RAITA *with* WARM PITA BREAD

Spring / Summer

Tamarind paste is produced from the fruit of the tamarind tree, a tropical leguminous tree that is thought to be native to Africa but today is grown in many other tropical regions. Tamarind is a sour pulp that is used widely across many traditional cuisines. It is also an ingredient in Worcestershire sauce, which gets quite a lot of use in my kitchen. In this recipe, the tamarind imparts a sticky, sharp tanginess to the chickpeas, which is in great contrast to the soothing raita.

Serves *2*
Time *30 minutes*

200 g (1 cup) cooked chickpeas or 1 x 400-g can chickpeas, rinsed and drained
1 tablespoon tamarind paste
1 teaspoon rapadura sugar
a knob of ginger, peeled and minced
extra-virgin olive oil
½ teaspoon cumin seeds
½ teaspoon coriander seeds
½ teaspoon mustard seeds, black or yellow
1 small red onion, thinly sliced
250 g (1 cup) coconut yoghurt, unsweetened (see page 254)
1 Lebanese or ½ continental cucumber, diced
a handful of fresh coriander, roughly chopped
fine salt
4 small whole wheat pita breads

Preheat the oven to 200°C.

Marinate the chickpeas in the tamarind, sugar and ginger by combining them in a bowl and leaving them to stand briefly while the oven comes up to temperature. When ready, spread the chickpeas out in a roasting dish and drizzle

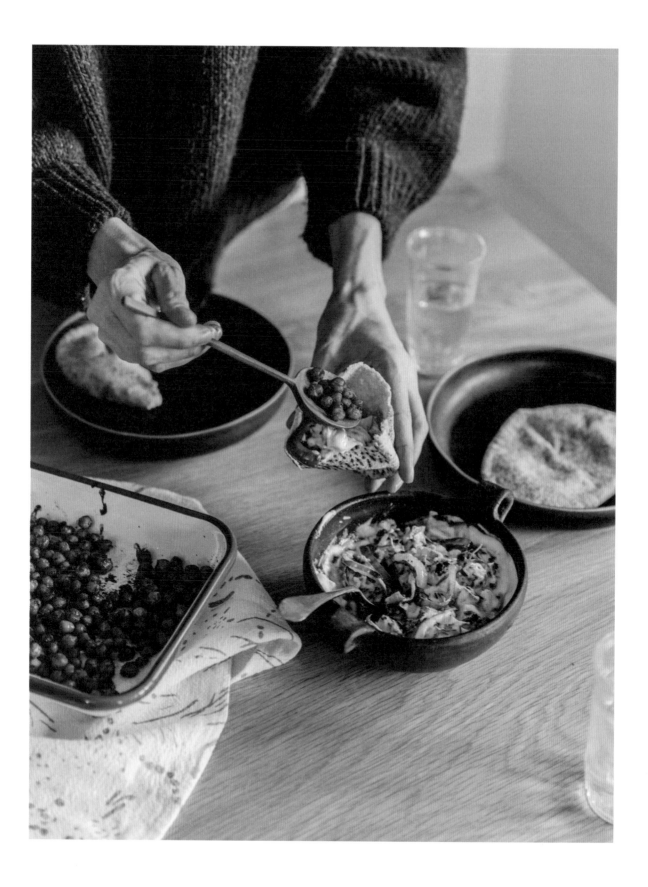

well with olive oil. Cook until crispy, about 20 minutes.

Warm a generous splash of olive oil in a frying pan over a medium heat. Briefly grind the spices with a mortar and pestle and add to the pan, along with the onion. Fry gently and stir regularly until the onion is soft, about 10 minutes, or longer if you prefer them crispy.

Meanwhile, combine the yoghurt, cucumber, coriander and a pinch of fine salt in a serving bowl. Top with the onion, pouring over any remaining oil and spices from the pan.

Remove the chickpeas from the oven, transfer to a serving bowl and season with salt. Heat the pita breads briefly in the still-warm oven or use a toaster.

To serve, halve each pita and cram in the raita and chickpeas.

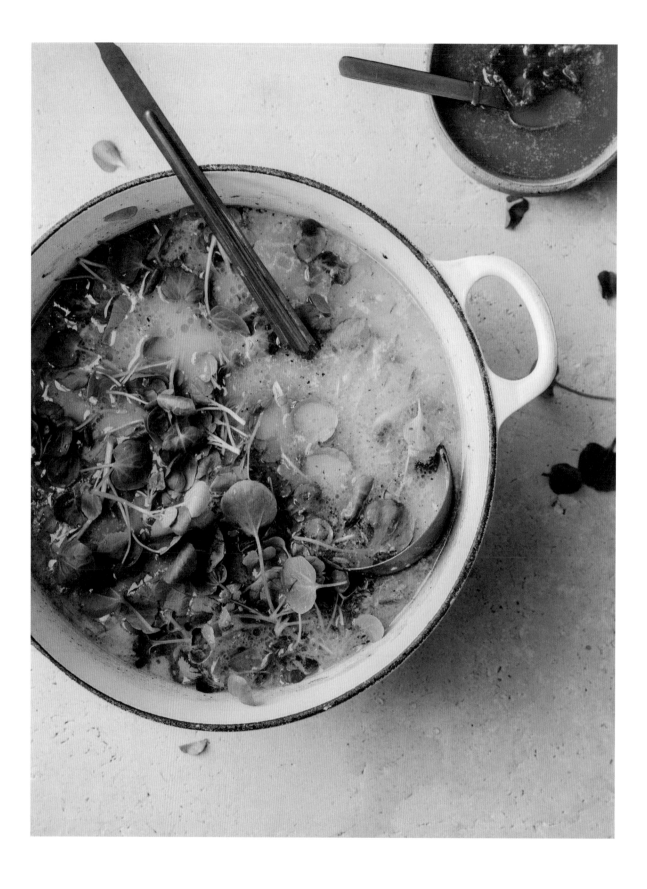

WATERCRESS *and* COCONUT SOUP *with* SUN-DRIED TOMATO *and* CHILLI OIL

Spring / Summer / Autumn
Gluten-free

In the first few weeks after giving birth, Bataknese women in the North Sumatra province of Indonesia eat torbangun soup three times a day.[168] Torbangun is the local name for *Coleus amboinicus*, which is known as Country or Indian borage in English. The word *bangun* translates to 'wake up' and is meant in the sense of giving strength to a mother. This restorative soup is made with several handfuls of leaves and coconut milk or water, and sometimes chicken or catfish as well.

This recipe is just as unassuming and laden with handfuls of nourishing watercress, but you can really use any greens you have to hand. If I were batch cooking this, I would only go so far as to make up the coconut broth. When needed, warm through a bowlful of broth and only add the fresh leaves just before eating, which will keep their colour, flavour and nutrients intact.

Serves *4 generously*
Time *45 minutes*

For the soup
extra-virgin olive oil
1 brown onion, diced
2 large zucchini (courgettes), topped and grated
400 ml (1½ cups + 1 tablespoon, or 1 x 400-ml can) coconut milk
875 ml (3½ cups) stock
juice of ½ a small lemon
ground black pepper
2 large handfuls of watercress, stems removed and roughly chopped

For the flavoured oil
40 g (¼ cup) sun-dried tomato strips
1 red chilli, deseeded and roughly chopped
185 ml (¾ cup) extra-virgin olive oil

Warm a generous splash of olive oil in a large saucepan over a medium heat. Sauté the onion and zucchini, stirring regularly, until the onion has softened, and the juices have started to release from the zucchini, about 10 minutes. Add the coconut milk, stock, lemon juice and season well with black pepper. Simmer, uncovered, until the onion is cooked through, about 20 minutes.

Meanwhile, prepare the flavoured oil by blending the sun-dried tomatoes, chilli and olive oil with a hand-held blender, until only small fragments of tomato and chilli remain, 3–4 minutes. At this point you can pour the oil through a sieve to create a smooth oil (compost the pulp or add to a chilli or similar), or you can keep it pulpy. To store any leftover flavoured oil, refrigerate it in an airtight container, like a jam jar. It should keep well for at least 6 months.

When the soup is ready, remove the pan from the heat and stir through the watercress, which will blanch cook in the residual heat. Use a hand-held blender to pulse into a thick and creamy soup, or keep the texture and silky leaves, by skipping this extra step.

Serve immediately with a drizzle of the flavoured oil.

CHIPOTLE BLACK BEANS
and MINCED WALNUTS *with* STOVETOP TOASTED CORN

Spring

Gluten-free

Weeknights for us, like many families, can be quite busy with afterschool activities and homework. Add in the general sense of exhaustion that can hit around 5 p.m. and there is little to no headspace for dinners that take an age to cook. I like this recipe because it comes together in half an hour, from pantry ingredients, and always goes down well with the boys. The secret is the chipotle — a dried jalapeño chilli pepper that is terrific at giving these beans an aged smokiness. They taste, in some magical way, like they have been on the stove all day. The first time you make this dish I would suggest erring on the side of caution and using the smaller amount of chipotle (¼ teaspoon), as I find a little of this piquant spice goes a long way. Along with the toasted corn, I would also serve this with crispy lettuce, and tortillas or rice.

Serves *4*
Time *30 minutes, plus soaking overnight*

For the chipotle beans
extra-virgin olive oil
1 brown onion, diced
120 g (1 cup) walnuts, soaked overnight and drained (see note)
4 cloves garlic
½ teaspoon ground cumin
¼–½ teaspoon ground chipotle
400 g (2 cups) cooked black beans or 2 cans, rinsed and drained
250 ml (1 cup) stock
250 ml (1 cup) passata
soy sauce

For the toasted corn
extra-virgin olive oil

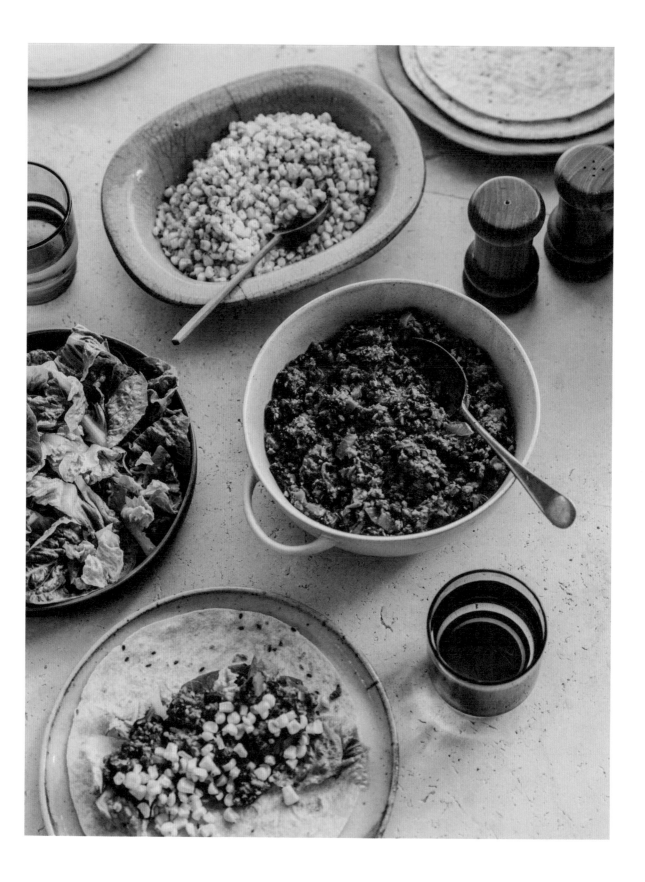

4 ears of fresh sweetcorn, kernels cut from the cob
ground black pepper
salt

To Serve
crispy lettuce
tortillas or rice

To make the chipotle beans

Warm a generous splash of olive oil in a large saucepan over a medium heat. Sauté the onion until soft and translucent, about 10 minutes.

Meanwhile pulse the walnuts and garlic briefly in a food processor to get a fluffy crumble consistency. Add to the pan with the cumin and chipotle and fry for a few minutes, stirring regularly, to toast the walnuts. Stir through the beans, stock, passata and a good splash of soy sauce. Heat to a simmer and cook until the sauce has reduced and thickened, about 20 minutes.

To make the toasted corn

Warm a generous splash of olive oil in a large frying pan over a medium heat. Sauté the sweetcorn, stirring regularly, until some of the kernels start to brown, about 10–15 minutes. Remove from the heat and season with salt and pepper.

To serve, warm the tortillas or rice on a plate and layer up with lettuce, beans and corn.

> NOTE
>
> *Many nuts can be processed to create a nut 'meat' that has a texture resembling minced/ground meat. Walnuts work particularly well in this regard, and I use them more this way than any other. The trick to making a good walnut meat is soaking the nuts well, ideally overnight, so that they have softened somewhat. Then pulse the nuts in a food processor so that they are fluffy and mince-like, without crunchy chunks, yet not ground so much that they start to get pasty.*

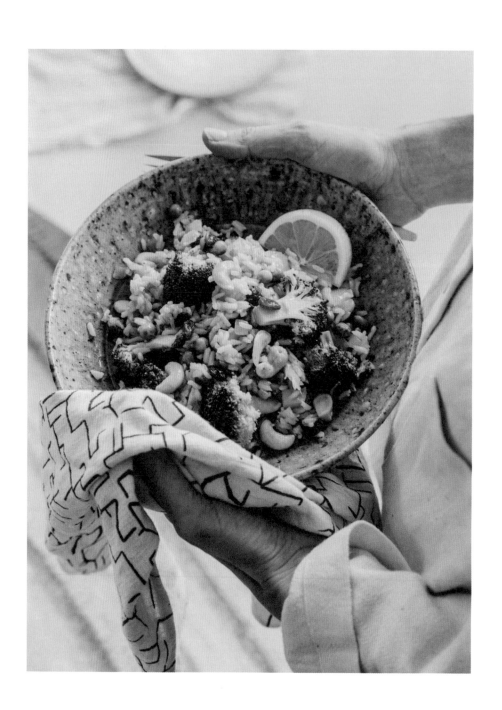

LEMONY BROCCOLI, PEA *and* GINGER BROWN RICE *with* TOASTED CASHEWS *and* STICKY SULTANAS

Spring / Autumn / Winter
Gluten-free

Stir-fries are my go-to for weeknight cooking. They are fast, flavourful and filling. This one is a favourite and simple to put together. I confess that if I'm tired I won't bother shelling fresh peas here. Rather, I'll toss them straight into the pan as they come — the pods will blister, and the steam will cook the peas inside out.

Serves *4*
Time *15 minutes*

300 g (1½ cups) long-grain brown rice, preferably soaked overnight
toasted sesame oil
extra-virgin olive oil
1 brown onion, diced
a knob of ginger, minced
80 g (½ cup) cashews, raw and unsalted
1 head of broccoli
a handful of freshly podded garden peas or 75 g (½ cup) frozen peas
80 g (½ cup) sultanas
1 tablespoon maple syrup or local honey
1 tablespoon tamari or soy sauce
1 unwaxed lemon, zested and then quartered
ground black pepper

Dry toast the brown rice in a saucepan for a few minutes, stirring well to prevent sticking. Add 625 ml (2½ cups) of just-boiled water, bring to a boil, then reduce to a simmer and cover and cook the rice until the water is absorbed, about 20 minutes. Turn off the heat and keep covered until ready to use.

Meanwhile, warm a generous splash of both oils in a large saucepan or wok over a medium heat. Add the onion, ginger and cashews, and sauté for a few minutes to soften the onion and toast the cashews a little.

Prepare the broccoli by chopping off the florets and dicing the stalk. Add to the pan with the onion along with the peas. Continue to sauté, stirring regularly to prevent sticking, but this time cover with a lid. Add more oil, if needed. Cook until the broccoli has blackened in places and the onion is brown, about 10 minutes.

Add the rice, sultanas, maple syrup (or honey), tamari (or soy), lemon zest and season well with black pepper. Cook uncovered over a low–medium heat, until the flavours are well combined, and the sultanas are warm and sticky, about 10 minutes.

Serve with wedges of lemon.

LENTIL, CHICKPEA *and*
BROWN RICE HARIRA

All seasons

Harira is a rich soup that originates from North Africa. It is traditionally eaten by Muslims during the holy month of Ramadan to break their fast at sunset. Being the sole meal eaten at this time, it is incredibly satisfying and nutritious. Harira is traditionally made with red meat stock, but vegetable stock will work or a combination of this and the broth from the canned chickpeas, if these are used. Harira means 'silk' in Arabic and the soup gets its velvety texture from the tedouira (meaning thickener), which is made separately and then poured into the main pot.

Serves *8*
Time *1 hour*

extra-virgin olive oil
1 brown onion, diced
a knob of ginger, peeled and minced
2 teaspoons cumin seeds
1 teaspoon harissa paste
1 teaspoon ground cinnamon
½ teaspoon ground turmeric
a pinch of saffron (optional)
ground black pepper
200 g (1 cup) or 1 x 400-g can cooked chickpeas, liquid reserved if using canned
   (see note)
150 g (¾ cup) long-grain brown rice, rinsed well
150 g (¾ cup) dried green lentils, rinsed well
1.5 litres (6 cups) stock

For the tedouira
125 g (½ cup) tomato paste
extra-virgin olive oil
35 g (¼ cup) white wheat flour, unbleached

a good pinch of salt
a handful of fresh coriander, finely chopped
a handful of fresh parsley, finely chopped

To serve
160 g (1 cup) pitted whole dates, roughly chopped
zest of 1 unwaxed lemon

Warm a generous splash of olive oil in a large saucepan over a medium heat. Add the onion and ginger and sauté for a few minutes to soften a little. Add the cumin, harissa, cinnamon, turmeric, saffron (if using), and season well with black pepper. Stir well to coat the onion with the spices. Add a little more olive oil if needed, so that the texture is like a paste. Add the chickpeas, rice, lentils and stock. Bring to a boil then reduce to a simmer and cook uncovered until the rice and lentils are cooked through, about 30 minutes. Stir regularly to prevent sticking.

Make the tedouira when the harira is nearly ready. In a separate saucepan, combine 500 ml (2 cups) water with the tomato paste and a splash of olive oil and bring to a boil. While coming to temperature, whisk the flour with 250 ml (1 cup) cold water in a separate jug or bowl, until it is all absorbed and milky. Take the tomato water off the heat, pour in the milky flour mix and a good pinch of salt, and whisk quickly to combine. Return the pan to the heat and cook until the tedouira is thickened and silky, about 2 minutes.

Add the tedouira, coriander and parsley to the main pot and stir to combine. Cook to allow the flavours time to come together, at least 20 minutes but longer if you have time.

Serve the harira in bowls topped with the chopped dates and lemon zest.

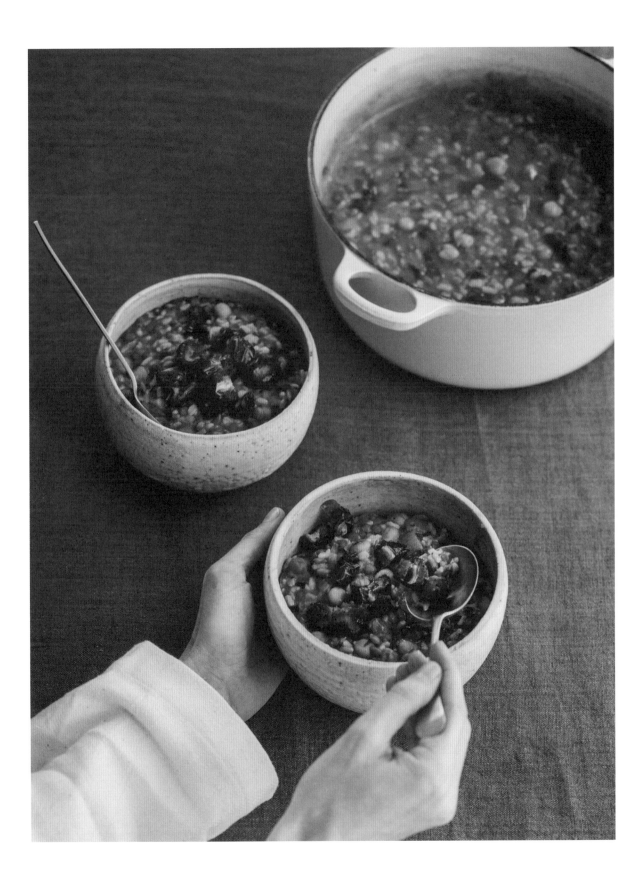

THREE SISTERS CHILLI

Spring / Summer / Autumn
Gluten-free

This dish feeds a crowd and is my go-to if we are having friends over for dinner. The recipe makes a thick and rich, tomatoey chilli that will be mild heat-wise. If you would like something hotter, add more fresh chilli or use cayenne, habanero, or chipotle in place of some of the smoked paprika. There is a special story behind the choice of ingredients (see overleaf).

Serves *8*
Time *2 hours*

extra-virgin olive oil
1 red onion, diced
4 cloves garlic, minced
1–2 jalapeño chilli peppers, deseeded and finely chopped
1 tablespoon cumin seeds
1 tablespoon ground coriander
1 tablespoon smoked paprika
1 litre (4 cups) stock
2 ears of fresh sweetcorn, kernels cut from the cob
300 g (2 cups) pumpkin, peeled, deseeded and cubed
400 g (3½ cups or 2 x 400-g cans, drained) cooked beans (see note)
215 g (1 cup) dried brown lentils
680 ml (4⅓ cups) passata

To serve
Rice, tortillas, tacos, nachos or baked potato
Cultured cashew cream (see page 257)

Warm a generous splash of olive oil in a large saucepan over a medium heat. Sauté the onion for a few minutes, stirring regularly, then add the garlic, chilli and spices, and cook until the onion is translucent and the spices are fragrant, about 5 minutes.

Add the stock and use a spatula to loosen any bits that have stuck to the base of the pan. Follow with the corn, pumpkin, beans and lentils. Bring to a boil and reduce

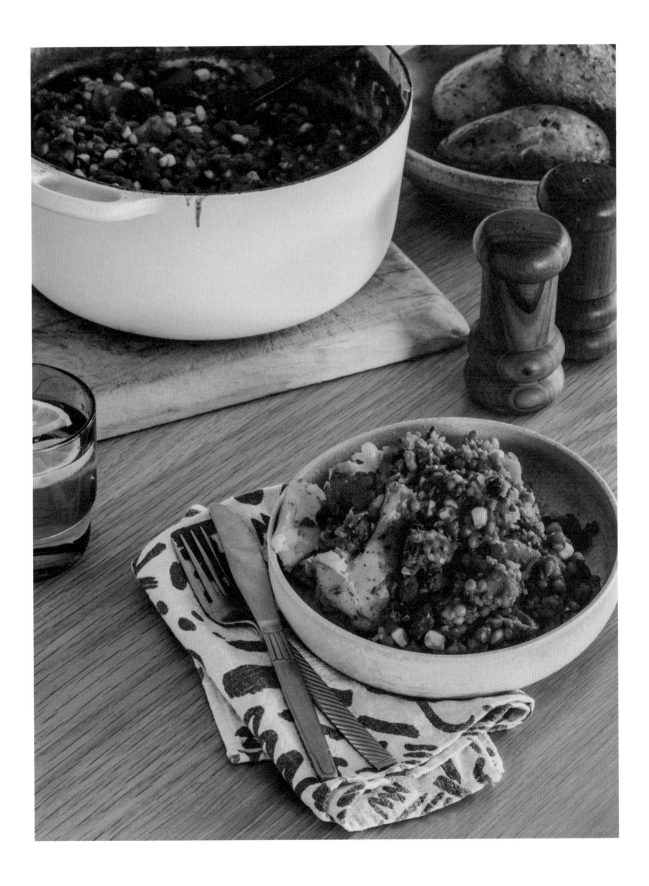

to a simmer. Cover and cook until the lentils and pumpkin have softened and most of the water has been absorbed, about 45 minutes. Stir occasionally to prevent sticking.

After this time, add passata and mash the pumpkin to thicken the sauce. Cook uncovered until the sauce has reduced and thickened further, about 45 minutes.

> NOTE
> *You can use soaked dried beans in place of canned beans but allow more stock. I like to use a mix of adzuki and black beans for this dish, but you could use any beans, or chickpeas would also work.*

The Three Sisters

For centuries before colonisation, the Three Sisters were central to the foodways of many Indigenous peoples of the Americas. The Three Sisters are three crops grown together — maize (corn), beans and squash/pumpkin — and are an example of an *inter(dependent) cropping* system, or companion planting, where the plants work together in ways that benefit each other.

The corn is planted first and as it matures it provides a sturdy vertical structure for the beans to climb. The beans are planted around the corn and draw nourishment into the soil from the nitrogen-fixing bacteria that live on the beans' roots. Lastly, the squash is planted around the corn and beans. The large leaves of the squash provide shade close to the ground, suppressing weeds, supporting water retention and preventing soil erosion.

When the Three Sisters are planted together, rather than as separate monocultures, they provide enough energy and protein per hectare to sustain around 13–16 people for a year, compared with 7–13 people when planted separately or in pairs.[169] For the women tending to the Three Sisters, the system was a sacred practice, imbued with culture, stories and ceremonies. As a reflection of corn's importance to their cultures, Native Americans incorporated corn into the names of many full moons, which marked the changing seasons — Planting Corn Moon, a Green Corn Moon, and a Moon When the Corn is in Silk.[170]

WHOLE ROOTS, BELUGA LENTIL *and* PINE NUT SALAD *with* MAPLE-MUSTARD DRESSING

All seasons

The leaves of many root vegetables are often forgotten but I show how you can celebrate them here in this colourful tray roast. The maple-mustard dressing is also a good recipe to have to hand — it will go well with any seasonal harvest salad.

Serves *4*
Time *1 hour 30 minutes*

For the salad
1 bunch (about 12) Dutch carrots, topped (tops reserved), tailed and scrubbed
1 bunch (about 10) baby beetroots, topped (leaves reserved), tailed, scrubbed and large ones halved
4 large potatoes, scrubbed and cubed
extra-virgin olive oil
salt
100 g (1 cup) beluga lentils, rinsed
root leaves (see page 44)
2 tablespoons pine nuts

For the dressing
60 ml (¼ cup) extra-virgin olive oil
2 tablespoons Dijon mustard
2 tablespoons maple syrup or local honey
1 tablespoon apple cider vinegar

Preheat the oven to 200°C.

Place the carrots, beetroot and potato in a large roasting dish, drizzle well with olive oil and add a good pinch of salt, and mix to coat. You may need to use two dishes to avoid crowding and to ensure even cooking. Roast until the vegetables are cooked and soft, about 1–1½ hours, tossing halfway through.

Meanwhile, simmer the lentils in 500 ml (2 cups) water, uncovered, until they

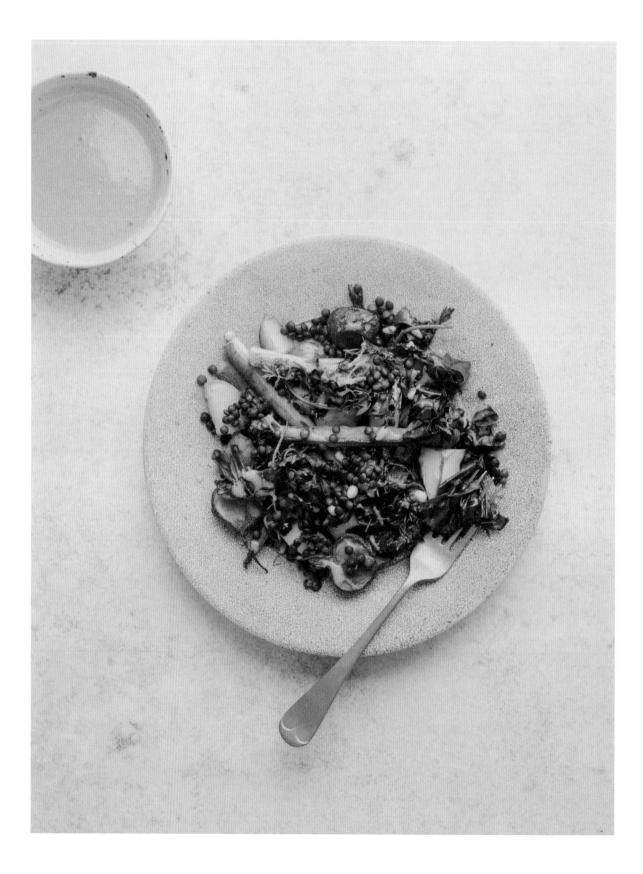

are soft and almost all of the water has been absorbed, about 30–40 minutes.

Prepare the dressing by whisking together the olive oil, mustard, maple syrup (or honey) and apple cider vinegar until well combined. Set aside.

Compost any root leaves that are bruised or well chewed by the bugs and place the rest along with the carrot tops and beet leaves into a sink full of water to loosen any soil and debris. Leave for at least 20 minutes or so, then drain the sink, rinse the leaves once more and roughly chop.

Warm a generous splash of olive oil in a large frying pan over a medium heat. Sauté the greens, stirring regularly, until the leaves have wilted, about 6–8 minutes. Add the pine nuts and cook for a few more minutes until they have toasted. Turn off the heat until the roast vegetables are ready.

Combine the roasted roots, lentils, greens and dressing, and mix well.

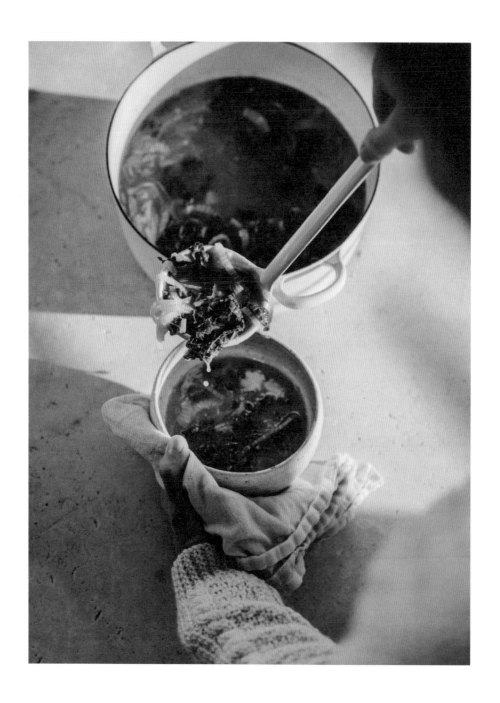

MISO, GINGER *and* BARLEY BROTH *with* WILTED GREENS

All seasons

This golden broth is a light meal but full of flavour. If you want to make this more substantial, add a drained can of chickpeas, or handful of dry toasted cashews. If you are making this ahead of time to freeze or refrigerate, follow all the steps but leave out the greens until you are ready to reheat. Wilted greens are best eaten warm and as close to fresh as possible, in my opinion.

Serves *4*
Time *1 hour*

extra-virgin olive oil
3 brown onions, halved and finely sliced
1 tablespoon maple syrup or local honey
4 cloves garlic, minced
a knob of ginger, peeled and minced
a good pinch of salt
150 g (¾ cup) pearled barley
1 bay leaf
1 tablespoon mugi miso
2 large handfuls of leafy greens, stems removed and roughly chopped, e.g. bok choi, silverbeet, kale

Warm a generous splash of olive oil in a large saucepan over a medium heat. Add the onion and maple syrup (or honey), and sauté, stirring regularly, until the onion is soft with some caramelised spots, about 20 minutes.

Add the garlic, ginger and a good pinch of salt, and sauté for a few minutes more to soften. Rinse the barley and add it to the pan, toasting it for a couple of minutes.

Add 2 litres (4 cups) boiled water and a bay leaf, and bring to the boil. Reduce the heat to a simmer, cover, and cook the broth until the barley has softened and cracked, about 30 minutes.

When the broth is ready, stir through the miso and place the leafy greens on top of the soup, cover, and steam for 10 minutes. Remove the bay leaf before serving.

COCONUT YOGHURT *and* LEMON DAHL *with* STICKY JASMINE RICE

All seasons
Gluten-free

Besides dahl, I cannot think of another meal that graces our table quite as often. There are infinite possibilities for adding flavour to a pot of thick, stewy lentils and I will never be done experimenting. This recipe is one of my favourites. Right until it is nearly ready, it fools you into thinking that it is nothing much to get excited about. But then the tangy yoghurt and rich tomato paste are added, and the dahl is transformed before your very eyes.

Serves *4*
Time *1 hour*

400 g (2 cups) jasmine rice, unrinsed
400 ml (1½ cups + 1 tablespoon) coconut milk
1 star anise (optional)
extra-virgin olive oil
1 brown onion, diced
2 cloves garlic, minced
a knob of ginger, peeled and minced
1 unwaxed lemon, zested and then quartered
1 teaspoon garam masala
1 teaspoon fenugreek seeds
300 g (1½ cups) split red lentils, rinsed well
1 litre (4 cups) stock
2 tablespoons tomato paste
2 tablespoons coconut yoghurt (see page 254)

Combine the rice, coconut milk, 250 ml (1 cup) water and the star anise, if using, in a saucepan. Bring to a boil then turn down the heat to a gentle simmer. Cover and cook for 20 minutes then turn off the heat and leave covered until ready to serve. Fluff with a fork and remove the star anise before serving.

Meanwhile, prepare the dahl. Warm a generous splash of olive oil in a large

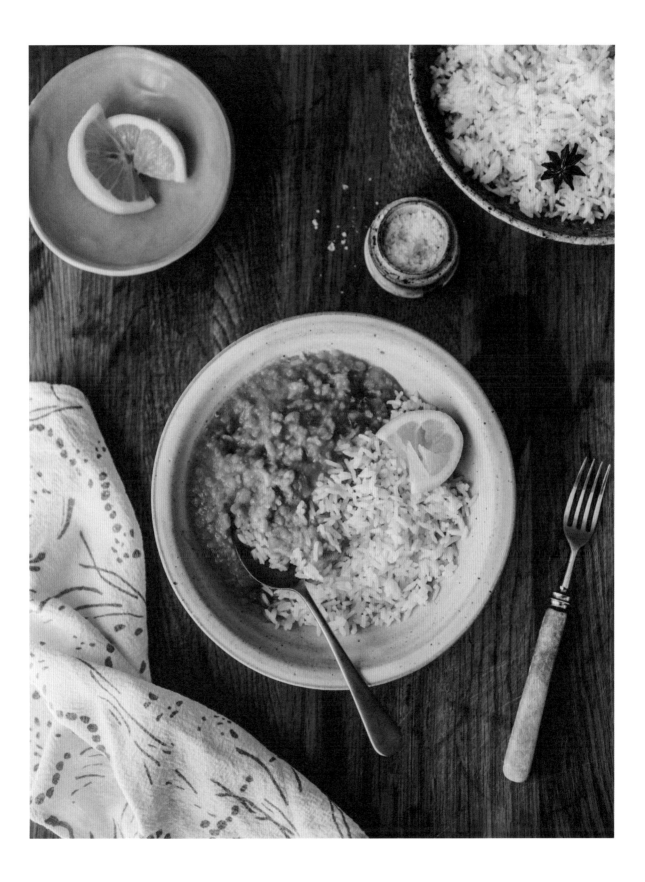

saucepan over a medium heat. Add the onion, garlic, ginger and lemon zest. Cook until the onion is soft and translucent, stirring regularly to prevent burning, about 10 minutes.

Add the garam masala and fenugreek and cook for a few minutes until they are fragrant. Then add the lentils and stock and bring to a boil. Turn down the heat to a gentle simmer. Cover and cook until the lentils have softened, about 30 minutes.

Stir through the tomato paste and coconut yoghurt, and cook for a few more minutes to bring the flavours together.

Serve the dahl with the rice and lemon wedges to the side.

ROAST POTATOES, CHERRY TOMATOES *and* SPROUTING BROCCOLI *with* CAPER PESTO

Spring/Summer/Autumn
Gluten-free

This is an unapologetically simple tray of roast potatoes dressed up with a vibrant pesto. I like to serve this as a side but if you'd like to make it more substantial, add some steamed green beans, pudgy butter beans or halved, soft- or hard-boiled eggs — there should be enough pesto to entertain any extra ingredients you like.

Serves *4*
Time *50 minutes*

800 g (3⅔ cups, about 4–5) potatoes, scrubbed and cubed
extra-virgin olive oil
500 g (2⅔ cups, 2 punnets) cherry tomatoes, halved
1 bunch of sprouting broccoli, thick stalks halved lengthways

For the pesto
40 g (¼ cup) pine nuts
3 large handfuls of fresh basil leaves
60 ml (¼ cup) extra-virgin olive oil
1 tablespoon salted capers, soaked and drained (see note)
juice of 1 small lemon
1 clove garlic, minced
ground black pepper

Preheat the oven to 200°C.

Spread the potatoes out in a roasting dish. Drizzle well with olive oil and cook in the oven for 20 minutes. Remove from the oven, add the cherry tomatoes and broccoli, drizzle with more olive oil and mix well. Return the dish to the oven and cook until potato is browned and cooked through, the tomatoes are soft and the broccoli slightly charred, about 20–30 minutes.

Meanwhile, to make the pesto, begin by dry toasting the pine nuts briefly in a

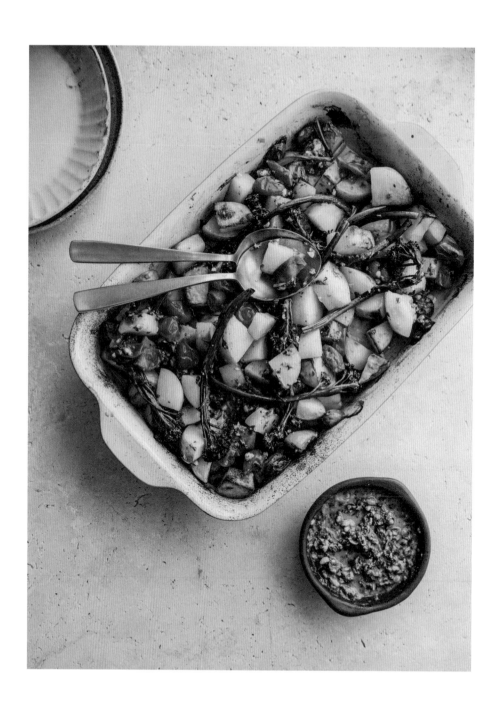

frying pan. Add these to the bowl attachment of a hand-held blender with the basil, olive oil, capers, lemon juice and garlic and season well with black pepper. Process into a thick paste, adding more oil if needed. Stir this into the vegetables when they are cooked through.

NOTE

Capers can be bought salted or in vinegar. The latter can be quite acidic, so I use salted here. To reduce their saltiness, soak the capers in warm water and drain. You may need to repeat this a couple of times until they don't taste salty anymore.

KALE, CANNELLINI *and* FARRO RIBOLLITA *with* SOURDOUGH

Spring / Winter

I was once fortunate enough to try a traditional ribollita on a day trip from Florence. I remember being sat outside on a terrace and gazing out across a quilted landscape of rolling hills, olive groves and Cyprus trees. The air was warm and the sunlight hazy. From behind his rustic, worn stone kitchen bench, the chef explained to me that ribollita means re-boiled in Italian. Leftover vegetable soup is layered between thick slices of stale bread and cooked for several hours to thicken. As he spoke, he gestured with his hands to show the layering of the ingredients. Ribollita is the ultimate peasant fare. It would have been made in huge pots and eaten for days on end, getting better each time — as soups most often do.

Serves *8–10*
Time *50 minutes to several hours*

extra-virgin olive oil
1 brown onion, diced
4 cloves garlic, minced
1 carrot, diced
1 stalk celery, diced
a handful of Tuscan kale (cavolo nero), stems removed and roughly chopped
150 g (2 cups) shredded Savoy or white cabbage
50 g (¼ cup) pearled farro, rinsed
200 g (1 cup or 1 x 400-g can) cannellini beans, rinsed and drained, stock reserved
1 large potato, scrubbed and cubed
2 litres (8 cups) stock
10 g (5 tablespoons) fresh thyme leaves, picked from stems
2 bay leaves
4 slices day-old whole wheat sourdough bread, each slice torn into 3 or 4 chunks

Warm a generous splash of olive oil in a large saucepan or stockpot over a medium heat. Sauté the onion, garlic, carrot and celery, stirring regularly, until the onion is soft and translucent, about 10 minutes.

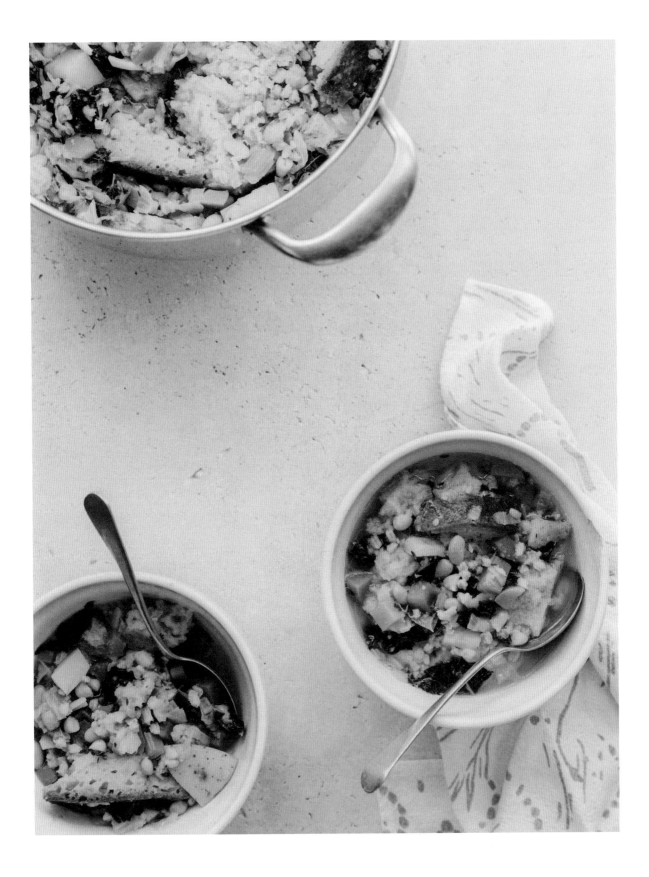

Add the kale, cabbage and farro and cook for a few minutes more to wilt the kale and toast the farro. Add the beans, potato, stock, thyme, bay leaves and a good slosh of olive oil.

Bring to a boil, then reduce to a simmer and cook, uncovered, until the farro has cooked through, about 40 minutes. At this point you can remove the bay leaves and enjoy the soup as it is or rest and re-boil it, as is traditionally done.

When ready to cook through a second time, ladle a third of the soup into a second large saucepan or stockpot. Arrange half of the bread in a layer across the soup. Repeat with another layer of soup, the last of the bread, and finish with a final layer of soup. Bring to a boil, then reduce to a simmer and cook, uncovered, until the bread has soaked into the soup and thickened it, about 20 minutes. Remove the bay leaves, if you haven't already done so, and serve.

PICKLED ONION *and* PUY LENTIL STEW *with* MASHED POTATO

All seasons

Gluten-free

As a child, every year at Christmas time we had a hamper delivered that contained all sorts of foods that we rarely, if ever, saw for the rest of the year. I would always be first into the giant box, digging around haphazardly, hoping to lay claim to the solitary jar of pickled onions before my siblings. I would eat them straight from the jar. They were sweet, crunchy and eye-wateringly acidic, and when I eat them now, I cannot help but be transported back to that time.

Another childhood food memory is my mother's stew. It was a hodgepodge of whatever was left in the cupboards, but always with barley. My mother would place the stew pot on the table next to a carefully constructed pyramid of sandwiches. We would help ourselves until we were stuffed; stew dribbling down our chins as we forgot our table manners and slurped every last drop from our bowls.

This stew is a portmanteau of these food memories. A sort of cross between a French onion soup and an Irish stew, but vegetable-based and with the potatoes on the side. Make sure to choose good-quality traditional pickled onions in malt vinegar. I find Puy lentils are great in stews — holding their shape and imparting a subtle peppery flavour. They are a protected cultivar — the champagne of lentils, if you like, grown only in the Le Puy area of France. If you would like to choose lentils that are locally grown, this recipe will not mind and I would encourage you to experiment, though I would keep to whole lentils rather than split.

Serves *6*
Time *1 hour 10 minutes*

For the stew
210 g (1 cup) Puy lentils
extra-virgin olive oil
150 g (about 8) pickled onions, drained and quartered
2 stalks celery, diced
2 carrots, halved lengthways and sliced

215

2 cloves garlic, minced

2 tablespoons flour

1¼ litres (5 cups) stock

1 tablespoon Worcestershire or soy sauce

10 g (5 tablespoons) fresh thyme leaves

1 bay leaf

a pinch of salt

ground black pepper

a handful of Tuscan kale (cavolo nero), stems removed and roughly chopped

2 tablespoons tomato paste

For the mashed potato

salt

1 kg (about 6 good-sized) potatoes, scrubbed or peeled, and cubed

extra-virgin olive oil

milk of your choice

6 spring onions, finely sliced

To make the stew

In a large saucepan, simmer the lentils in 750 ml (3 cups) water until they are soft, and all the water has been absorbed, about 20 minutes.

Warm a generous splash of olive oil in a large saucepan over a medium heat. Sauté the pickled onion, celery, carrot and garlic, stirring regularly, until the onion has started to brown, about 15–20 minutes. Meanwhile, prepare the potatoes (below).

Add the flour to stew ingredients, stir well to coat, and sauté for a few minutes. Follow with the stock, Worcestershire or soy sauce, thyme and bay leaf, and season well with salt and pepper.

Simmer to thicken the stew and combine the flavours, about 20 minutes. Finally, add the cooked lentils, kale and tomato paste and cook through, about 10 minutes.

To make the mashed potato

Bring a large saucepan of salted water to a boil, add the potatoes and reduce to a simmer. Cook, uncovered, until the potatoes slide freely off an inserted knife, about 20 minutes.

Drain the potatoes and return to the pan. Add a splash of olive oil and enough milk so that when mashed, the potato is creamy and soft. Stir through the spring onion.

To serve, plate the mash and top with a generous spoonful of stew.

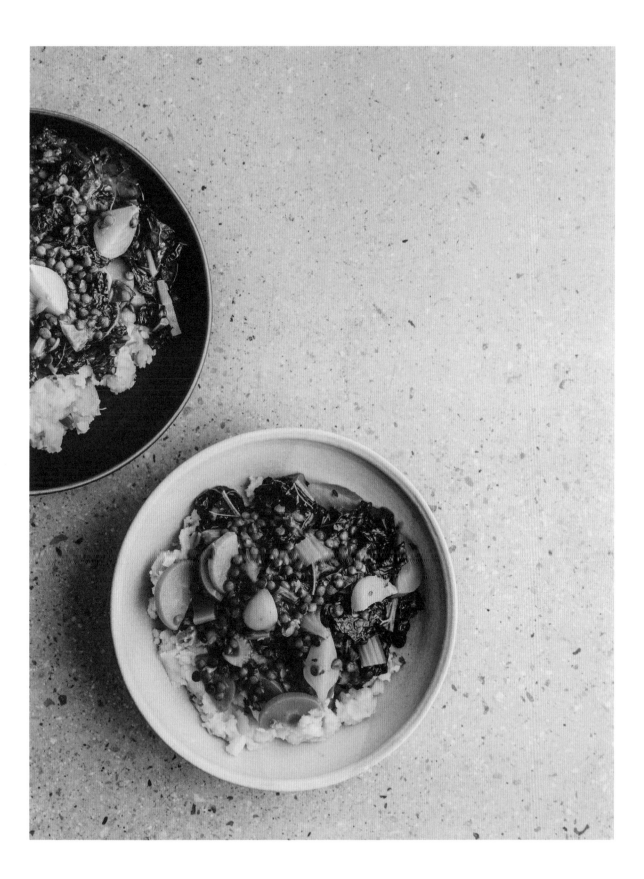

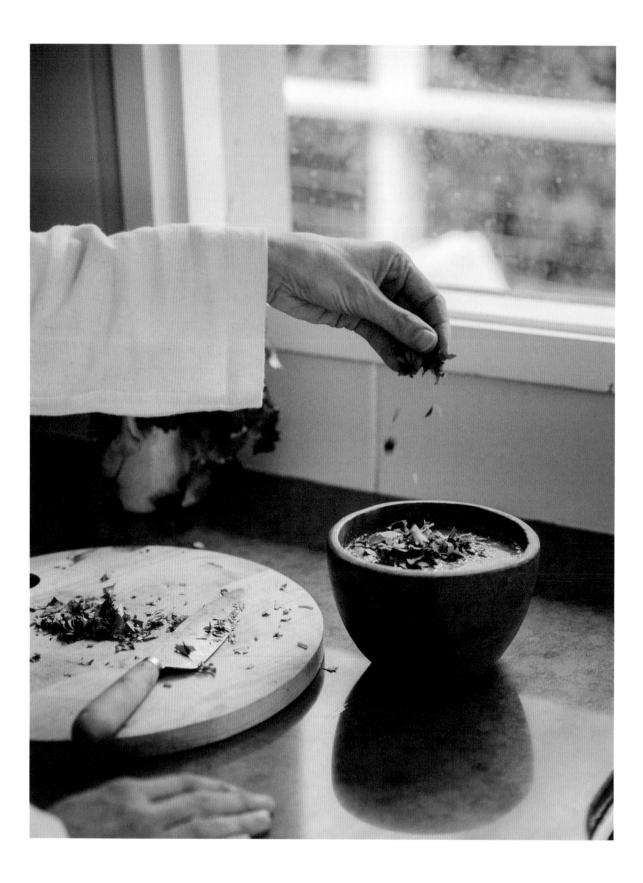

QUINOA, POTATO *and* CORN SOUP *with* SWEET YELLOW CHILLI

Spring
Gluten-free

Quinoa soup is often eaten by Andean women in the postpartum period, as it is believed to promote the production of breast milk. This recipe is my version of this traditional practice. It is quite substantial like a chowder, but still brothy and hydrating. I use potatoes and corn, which are staple ingredients in Andean cuisine, as well as a paste made from a sweet hot yellow chilli that is grown in Peru, called Aji Amarillo. I have been unable to source this chilli fresh in Australia, although you can get the paste from speciality food stores and online. It is worth trying to get hold of a jar as it is very delicious and a little goes a long way. You can use the smallest amount to add heat to curries, chillies and the like. As an alternative here, I have used a sweet banana chilli and ground cayenne, which are more readily available. Traditionally, the soup often contains the meat from a local bird called a Flicker, and you may like to use chicken stock and add in some shredded chicken meat, in a similar fashion.

Serves *4*
Time *40 minutes*

extra-virgin olive oil
1 brown onion, diced
1 stalk celery, finely chopped
2 cloves garlic, minced
100 g (½ cup) quinoa, rinsed well
½–1 teaspoon Aji Amarillo paste or 1 sweet yellow chilli (banana chilli), finely
   sliced and ¼ teaspoon ground cayenne pepper (cayenne optional)
1.5 litres (6 cups) stock
400 g (about 2) potatoes, scrubbed and cubed
1 ear of fresh sweetcorn, kernels cut from the cob
a handful of fresh coriander, finely chopped
ground black pepper

Warm a generous splash of olive oil in a large saucepan over a medium heat. Add the onion, celery and garlic, and sauté over a low–medium heat, stirring regularly, until the onion has softened, about 10 minutes.

Add the quinoa and the chilli paste (or chilli and cayenne, if using) and toast the quinoa, stirring regularly for a few minutes. Add the stock, potato and corn, bring to a boil, then reduce to a simmer, covered, until the potato is soft, and the quinoa is cooked through, about 20–25 minutes.

Stir through the coriander and season well with black pepper just before serving.

WILD GREENS, LEEK *and* CULTURED CASHEW CREAM TART *with* MARJORAM

All seasons

It is always good to have on hand a pastry recipe that can work with any manner of fillings. Here she is filled with wild greens, but you could try roast beetroot, or pumpkin and sage as well. The honey and mustard in the crust give just a subtle hint of sunshine. I like to serve this with a couple of new potatoes and a heap of garden peas, but it also packs up well for a picnic. If you don't have any cashew cream to hand, ricotta would make a good substitute.

Makes *1 tart to serve 4–6*
Time *1 hour 40 minutes*

For the pastry
250 g (1⅔ cups) whole wheat flour
1 tablespoon ground flaxseeds (linseeds)
1 tablespoon ground mustard
a good pinch of fine salt
80 ml (⅓ cup) extra-virgin olive oil
1 tablespoon local honey or maple syrup

For the filling
extra-virgin olive oil
1 leek, finely chopped
2 large handfuls (400 g) wild leafy greens, e.g. rocket (arugula), dandelion,
    nettle, finely chopped
2 cloves garlic, minced
a small handful of fresh marjoram leaves, picked from stems, plus extra to serve
1 quantity cultured cashew cream (see page 257), or 230 g (1 cup) ricotta
juice of a small lemon
a pinch of salt
ground black pepper
1 tablespoon pine nuts
local honey or maple syrup

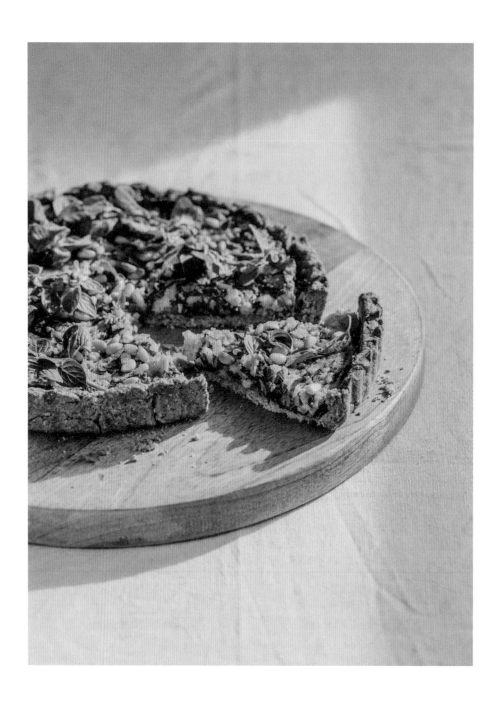

To make the pastry

Preheat the oven to 180°C. Grease a 24-cm loose-bottomed tart tin. Place a jug with 80 ml (⅓ cup) water in the freezer.

In a large bowl, whisk the flour, flaxseeds, mustard and salt until well combined. Add the olive oil and honey (or maple syrup) and stir until the mix becomes crumbly. Use the tips of your fingers to gently break up the mixture until the texture resembles evenly sized breadcrumbs. Bring the water out of the freezer and slowly add it to the mix. As you add the water, knead the dough to bring it together. When the dough holds in a tacky ball, stop adding the water — you may not need to use it all.

Transfer the dough to a clean work surface and knead until it is soft and supple, but still with a few cracks, about 5 minutes. Return to the bowl and cover with a damp tea towel. Refrigerate for 10 minutes.

Still on a clean work surface, roll out the pastry to the thickness of a coin in a circle a little wider than the tart tin. Transfer the pastry to the tin and push it gently into the edges, leaving a slight overhang. Prick the base of the pastry case really well all over with a fork.

Line the tart tin with baking parchment and fill with ceramic baking beans, dried pulses or rice. Bake until the pastry is firm, about 20 minutes, then remove the beans. Trim off any excess pastry using a small, serrated knife and cook until golden on the base, about 10 minutes more.

To make the filling

Warm a generous splash of olive oil in a large frying pan over a medium heat. Sauté the leek, stirring regularly, until sweet and soft, about 10 minutes. Add the leafy greens, garlic and marjoram and cook for a few minutes to wilt the leaves. Stir through the cashew cream (or ricotta) and lemon juice and season with salt and pepper.

Spoon the filling into the tart case and spread to the edges. Sprinkle the pine nuts over the top and drizzle with a little honey (or maple syrup).

Bake until completely cooked through and the pine nuts have toasted a little, about 30 minutes. Serve with a scattering of fresh marjoram leaves.

SUN-DRIED TOMATO *and* PESTO MUFFINS *with* PEPITAS

All seasons

A really good muffin recipe is always worth knowing. These are a savoury version — soft and light and packed with flavour from sun-dried tomatoes and pesto. I often make these to pop into lunchboxes or to take on day trips to the beach, as they travel so well. Use any pesto you like in this recipe, homemade or good-quality shop-bought.

Makes *12 muffins*
Time *30 minutes*

150 g (1 cup) whole wheat flour
150 g (1 cup) white flour, unbleached
2 tablespoons ground flaxseeds (linseeds) or 2 eggs, beaten
2 teaspoons baking powder, aluminium-free
1 teaspoon sweet paprika
a pinch of fine salt
150 ml (½ cup + 1 tablespoon) extra-virgin olive oil
330 ml (1⅓ cups) milk of your choice, plus extra to brush the muffin tops
75 g (½ cup) sun-dried tomato strips, roughly chopped
1 carrot, grated
90 ml (⅓ cup) pesto (good-quality shop-bought or see page 209)
pepitas to decorate

Preheat the oven to 180°C. Line a 12-cup muffin tin with paper cases.

Combine the flours, flaxseed, baking powder, paprika and salt in a large bowl and mix well. If using an egg in place of flaxseeds, add this with the wet ingredients (the olive oil and milk).

Stir in the olive oil, milk, sun-dried tomato and carrot. Loosely swirl through the pesto, keeping streaks visible. Spoon the batter into the cases, sprinkle with pepitas and brush with milk.

Bake the muffins until cooked through and golden and a skewer inserted into the centre comes out clean, about 30 minutes. Transfer to a cooling rack and cool before eating.

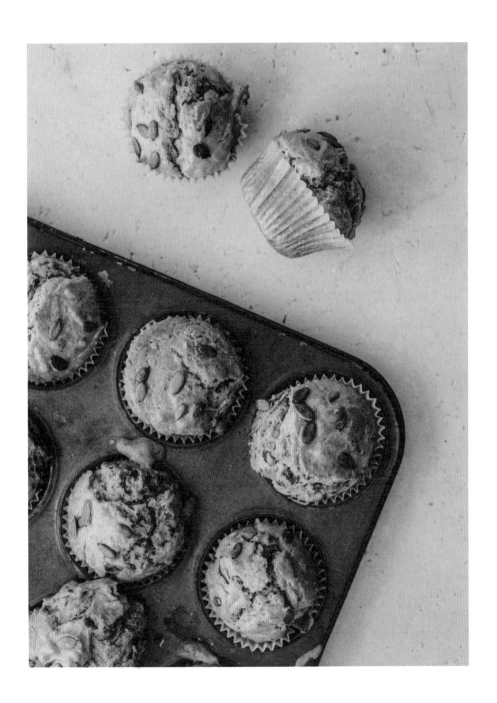

DATE *and* PECAN SCONES *with* GINGER

All seasons

If you are wanting something warming for morning or afternoon tea, these scones are perfect. Caramelly dates and buttery pecans go so well with the spiced, flaky dough (note that the large amount of cinnamon is not a typing error). Enjoy these soon after they are ready, with a hot drink and good conversation.

Makes *about 8 scones*
Time *45 minutes*

90 g (½ cup) pitted dried dates, chopped
200 g (1⅓ cups) whole wheat flour, plus extra for dusting
70 g (⅓ cup) rapadura sugar
1 tablespoon ground flaxseeds (linseeds)
1 tablespoon ground cinnamon
1 teaspoon ground ginger
1 teaspoon baking powder, aluminium-free
80 ml (⅓ cup) extra virgin coconut oil, melted and cooled
125 ml (½ cup + 1 tablespoon) milk of your choice
50 g (½ cup) whole pecans, chopped, plus extra for topping

Preheat the oven to 180°C. Line a baking tray with parchment paper.

Soak the dates in boiled water until soft, about 10 minutes, then drain.

Meanwhile, combine the flour, sugar, flaxseed, cinnamon, ginger and baking powder in a large bowl and mix well.

Cut in the coconut oil by using your fingers to rub it into the flour until you have a fine crumb. Pour in the milk and bring the dough together with your hands. Lastly, knead in the dates and pecans and leave for a few minutes for the dough to rest.

Empty the dough into a mound on the baking tray. Dust the top with flour and pat down gently to spread out into a round (called a 'bannock' in Scotland), until the dough is about the thickness of your thumb. Press a few pecans into the top of the dough.

Bake until cooked through, about 20 minutes. Cut into wedges while warm.

CARDAMOM *and* BROWN RICE KHEER *with* HONEYED PLUMS

Summer / Autumn
Gluten-free

Kheer is a traditional Indian pudding made with basmati rice and milk. The word kheer comes from the Sanskrit word for a dish prepared with milk, *kshirika*. According to ancient Indian texts, kheer or *payasam*, as it is also known, is a dish that is recorded as being eaten since ancient times. It is mentioned in Ayurveda (an ancient system of medicine) and many traditional cultures have their own rice pudding recipes that are alike in their simplicity.

As a child, my mother would sometimes give us a simple rice pudding made with short-grain rice, milk, cream and sugar. This recipe reminds me of that. I would serve this after a light dinner such as dahl or on its own as a tide-over between meals. Kheer feels particularly nourishing when convalescing or when you have a small appetite, as it goes down effortlessly. I have suggested a quick honeyed plum recipe to add a sharp, sweet contrast, but any fresh or dried fruit and some chopped nuts will go well.

Serves *4*
Time *40 minutes*

For the kheer
extra-virgin coconut oil
3–4 green cardamom pods
200 g (1 cup) brown basmati rice, preferably soaked overnight
1 litre (4 cups) milk of your choice
35 g (¼ cup) shelled pistachios, roughly chopped, to serve

For the plums
1 tablespoon extra-virgin coconut oil
1 tablespoon local honey or maple syrup
2 plums, halved and stones removed
a good pinch of ground cinnamon

To make the kheer

Warm a teaspoon of coconut oil in a large saucepan over a medium heat. Crush the cardamom pods, compost the green outer layer and empty the inner black seeds into the pan. Follow with the rice and toast together with the seeds for a few minutes until fragrant.

Pour in the milk and bring to a boil, watching the pan carefully so it does not spill over. Reduce the heat to a simmer, then cover and cook the rice until soft, about 20 minutes. When the rice is cooked, keep the lid on and leave to stand and thicken a little, about 10 minutes. Remove any skin before serving.

To make the plums

Warm the coconut oil and honey (or maple syrup) in a frying pan over a medium heat until small bubbles appear. Meanwhile, slice each of the plums into 16 or so segments. Add the cinnamon to the pan and swirl the ingredients together. Follow with the plum segments. Fry the plums until they are honey yellow and soft, then flip over and repeat on the other side, about 4 minutes each side.

To serve, spoon some warm kheer into a bowl, top with honeyed plums and sprinkle over the chopped pistachios.

BUTTERMILK BROWNIES
with CASHEW CARAMEL

All seasons

These brownies involve a little groundwork. There is chocolate to melt, buttermilk to make and flaxseeds to thicken. However, the end result is soft and rich, with a flaky, crackled top — absolutely worth the extra washing up. They are delicious on their own, but if you'd like to indulge (and why not?), I have included a handy recipe for a cashew caramel sauce to drizzle over when they are cooling.

Makes *9 brownies*
Time *40 minutes*

For the brownies
80 g (½ cup) fair trade dark chocolate
125 ml (½ cup) milk of your choice
1 tablespoon lemon juice or apple cider vinegar
1 teaspoon vanilla essence
1 tablespoon ground flaxseeds (linseeds)
100 g (⅔ cup) whole wheat flour
2 tablespoons rapadura sugar
½ teaspoon bicarbonate of soda
a pinch of fine salt
145 ml (½ cup + 1 tablespoon) extra-virgin olive oil, mild flavour

For the caramel
2 tablespoons rapadura sugar
1 tablespoon cashew butter
1 tablespoon boiled water

To make the brownies
Preheat the oven to 180°C. Grease and line a 20-cm square cake tin with parchment paper.

Melt the chocolate in a double boiler — fill a saucepan a quarter full with water that has just boiled in a kettle. Keep the water simmering over a low–medium heat

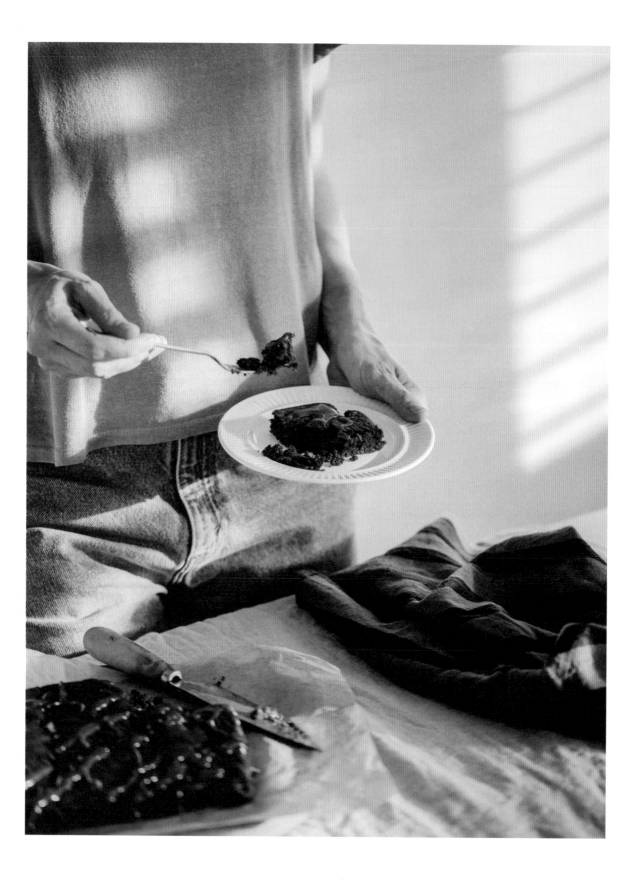

and place a large bowl on top of the pan. Break up the chocolate into the bowl and let the steam on the base of the bowl gently melt the chocolate. Turn off the heat when there are no chunks visible, about 5 minutes.

Meanwhile, make the buttermilk in a small jug or mug. Combine the milk, lemon juice (or vinegar) and vanilla and stir well. Set aside until clumpy, about 5 minutes.

In another small jug or mug, whisk the flaxseeds and 2½ tablespoons water. Leave to thicken, about 5 minutes.

Combine the flour, sugar, bicarbonate of soda and salt in a mixing bowl and make a well in the centre. Pour the olive oil, melted chocolate and the prepared flaxseeds and buttermilk, into the centre of the well. Use a metal spoon or spatula to beat the wet ingredients together until smooth and then continue outwards to gently fold in the dry ingredients just enough until there is no flour visible.

Pour the batter into the prepared baking tin and, if needed, use the back of the spoon or spatula to spread the batter into the corners of the tin.

Bake the brownie until cooked through and a skewer inserted into the centre yields a few crumbs, about 20 minutes. Meanwhile make the caramel (see below).

Leave the brownie in the tin for a few minutes, then lift out onto a cooling rack using the edges of the baking paper. The brownie may crack on top when you do this, which is all the better as it creates furrows to catch the caramel. Use a knife to cut the brownie into 9 squares.

To make the caramel

Place the sugar in a small pan and use your fingers to sprinkle a few drops of water into it until it resembles wet sand then set aside.

Make a cream with the cashew butter and boiled water by whisking them together in a small bowl until smooth and well combined.

Warm the pan over a medium heat until the sugar melts to look and smell like treacle and small bubbles appear at the edges. Immediately remove from the heat and hastily whisk in the cashew cream to create the caramel. Drizzle over the cooked brownie.

NOTES
Depending on the quality of the cashew butter, some caramels may seem a little gritty from small bits of nuts that were not blitzed enough. This is okay, but if you would prefer a silkier caramel, push the caramel through a tea strainer or sieve using the back of a spoon.

POACHED PEAR *and* PRUNE CRUMBLE *with* ALMONDS *and* DARK CHOCOLATE

Summer / Autumn / Winter

Crumbles are a super way to use up and enjoy a glut of seasonal fruit. This whole wheat, olive oil and almond topping will work with any filling. In this case I have used pears, but apples, or stewed rhubarb, berries or stone fruit would also go well. The pears and prunes in this recipe are excellent to support gut motility — a delicious way to move things along if you are feeling sluggish.

Serves *8*
Time *50 minutes*

4 pears, peeled, halved lengthways and cored
125 g (½ cup) pitted prunes, chopped
1 teaspoon ground cinnamon or 1 cinnamon stick
1 star anise (optional)
150 g (1 cup) whole wheat flour
70 g (⅓ cup) rapadura sugar
100 ml (½ cup + 1 tablespoon) extra-virgin olive oil, light flavour
80 g (½ cup) almonds, roughly chopped
50 g (½ cup) rolled oats
35 g (¼ cup) dark chocolate, broken into chunks

Preheat the oven to 180°C. Place the pears, prunes, cinnamon and star anise, if using, in a saucepan and cover with water. Bring to a boil then turn down the heat and simmer until the pears are soft, about 10 minutes.

Combine the flour, sugar and oil in a bowl and rub the ingredients into an even crumble consistency. Stir through the almonds and oats.

Use a slotted spoon to remove the pears and prunes from the pan and transfer them into an ovenproof dish. Carefully pour over a little of the poaching liquid and then top with the crumble mix. Sprinkle over the chocolate and bake until cooked through and piping hot, about 20 minutes.

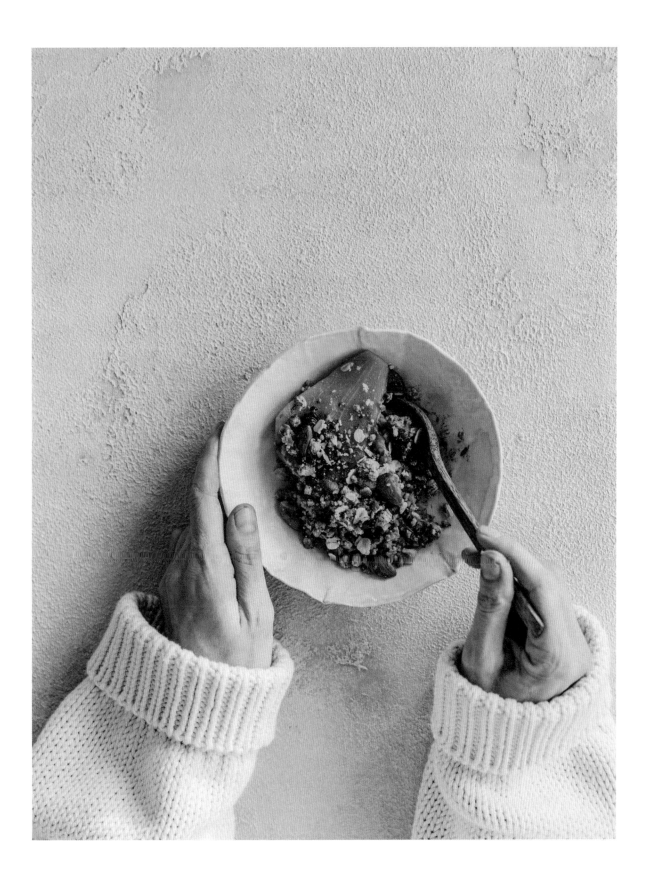

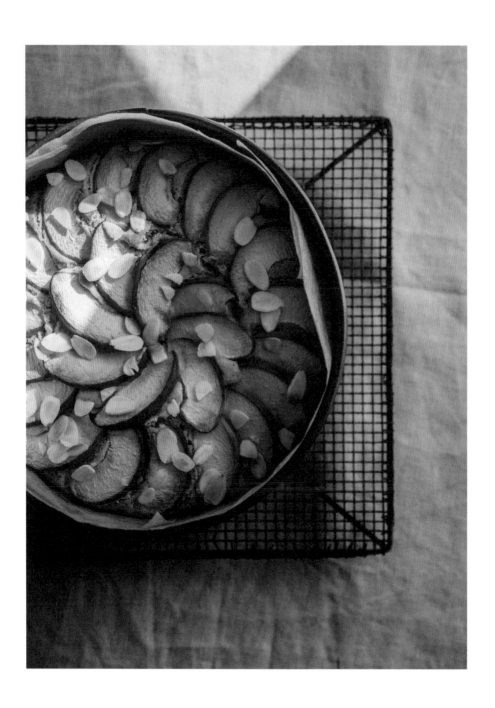

PEACH, HONEY *and* SEMOLINA CAKE *with* ALMONDS

Summer / Autumn

Every mother is in need of one simply made, beautiful cake for celebrations, and this is she. Golden yellow, sweet and soft, and a perfect cushion for the peaches. The lemon juice keeps the colour of the peaches, so don't skip this step.

Serves *8–10*
Time *40 minutes*

2 tablespoons ground flaxseeds (linseeds)
1 ripe yellow peach, halved and pitted
juice of 1 lemon
180 g (1 cup) finely milled semolina/durum flour
150 g (1 cup) white wheat flour, unbleached
1 teaspoon baking powder, aluminium-free
½ teaspoon bicarbonate of soda
170 ml (⅔ cup) extra-virgin olive oil, mild flavour
175 g (½ cup) lightly flavoured local honey or maple syrup
170 ml (⅔ cup) milk of your choice
35 g (¼ cup) flaked almonds

Mix the flaxseed with 80 ml (⅓ cup) water in a small bowl and set aside. Finely slice the peach and toss in a bowl with the lemon juice, then set aside.

Preheat the oven to 180°C. Grease and line a 23-cm round loose-bottomed or springform cake tin.

In a large bowl, combine the semolina, flour, baking powder and bicarbonate of soda. Make a well in the centre and pour in the olive oil, honey (or maple syrup) and milk. Fold the ingredients together until no flour is visible and the batter is smooth.

Pour the batter into the cake tin and arrange the peaches in a spiral, beginning from the outside and working inwards, gently pressing them into place. Sprinkle the flaked almonds on top.

Bake until the cake is golden, and a skewer inserted into the centre comes out clean, about 30 minutes. Allow it to cool a little in the pan and then transfer to a rack.

GINGER TEA *and* MELON ICE BLOCKS

Spring/Summer

The ginger tea in these ice blocks makes them zingy and refreshing — they are excellent if you are suffering from morning sickness. If you wanted a version for the cooler months, you could try fresh orange in place of the melon, just be sure to remove any pips.

Makes *about 8 ice blocks*
Time *20 minutes plus 12 hours freezing*

a knob of fresh ginger, sliced
1 small lemon, finely sliced
1 tablespoon local honey or maple syrup
½ rockmelon (cantaloupe), peeled, deseeded and chopped

Steep the ginger and lemon slices in 500 ml (2 cups) boiled water in a saucepan or large jug. After 10 minutes, drain the tea and compost the ginger and lemon. Stir through the honey (or maple syrup). When cool, transfer to a food processor together with the melon and blitz to get a pulpy consistency. Pour into ice block moulds and freeze overnight.

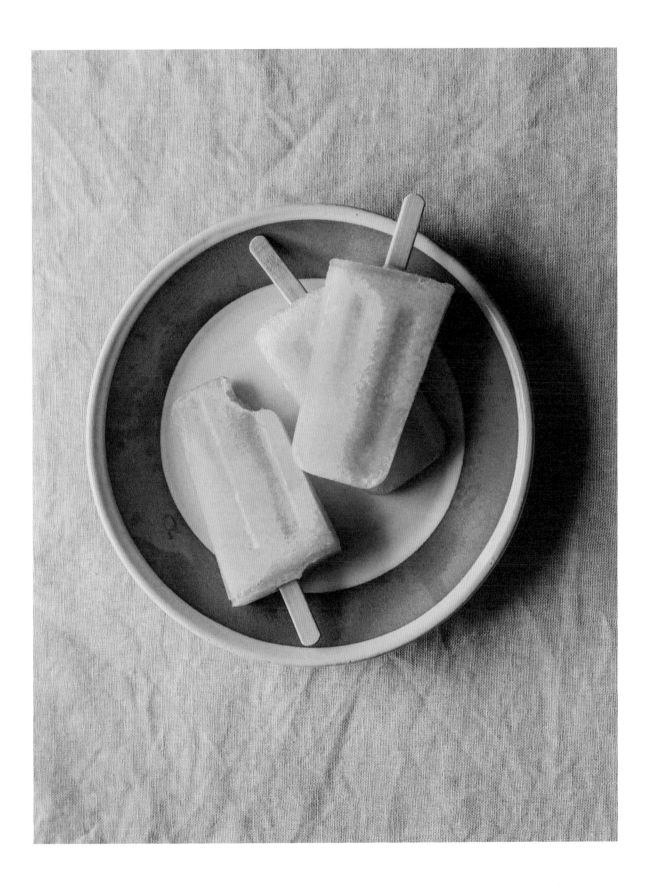

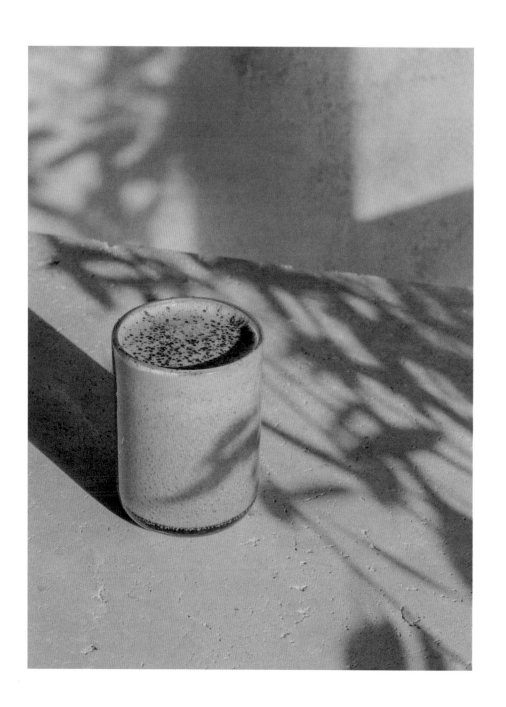

CHOCOLATE *and* CASHEW SHAKE

All seasons
Gluten-free

If you have a powerful blender, then use plump whole prunes for this quick, creamy shake, but if not, prune juice will give a smoother texture. This can be served cold like a milkshake or warmed through on the stove (or using a milk steamer, if you have one) as a hot chocolate.

Serves *1–2*
Time *5 minutes*

310 ml (1¼ cups) milk of your choice, chilled
60 ml (¼ cup) prune juice or 4 prunes, pitted
2 tablespoons cashew butter
1½ teaspoons cocoa or cacao (see note)
a pinch of ground cinnamon
local honey or maple syrup to taste

Combine all the ingredients in a high-speed blender and process until smooth and creamy. Taste and add a little honey (or maple syrup) if you like, and pulse again to combine.

NOTE

Although cocoa and cacao are spelled similarly, there are differences between these ingredients. Both come from cacao pods — large sacks of pulpy seeds that grow on the cacao tree. These cacao 'beans' are bitter and astringent but are transformed through several days of fermenting and drying. At this point, the dry cacao beans can be ground into a meal, which is available in the shops as raw cacao powder. Or the beans head to factories, where they are roasted and ground to produce cocoa powder.

Dutched or alkalised cocoa goes through a further process to change its pH and produce a milder flavour. This extra processing step substantially reduces the amount of beneficial antioxidant compounds the cocoa contains.[171]

If you would like to avoid any of the stimulating compounds found in cocoa or cacao, then carob is worth trying. Carob is a legume that grows on trees as long seed-containing pods, which are dry-roasted and milled to make a flour. It contains no caffeine or theobromine.

Choose ethically sourced (independently certified) cacao products, including chocolate. Unfortunately, modern-day slavery is not uncommon in cacao supply chains.

WHOLE WHEAT CRACKERS
and DULSE *with* ZA'ATAR

All seasons

Za'atar is a Middle Eastern spice mix. Traditionally, its base would contain toasted sesame seeds, Syrian oregano, salt and sumac — the ground drupes of the sumac tree — but there are countless versions available. Za'atar has many uses, not least as a dip, sprinkle or rub. If you would like to make a plainer version of these crackers, you can do so by omitting the za'atar. Alternatively, you could replace it with some mixed herbs or finely grated hard cheese like Parmesan or Pecorino.

Makes *about 40 crackers*
Time *30 minutes*

185 g (1¼ cups) whole wheat flour
2 tablespoons ground flaxseeds (linseeds)
2 tablespoons za'atar
2 teaspoons rapadura sugar
2 teaspoons dried dulse flakes (see note)
a pinch of fine salt
80 ml (⅓ cup) extra-virgin coconut oil, melted and cooled
60 ml (¼ cup) water
black sesame seeds to garnish

Preheat the oven to 180°C.

In a large bowl, combine the flour, flaxseeds, za'atar, sugar, dulse and salt, and mix well. Add the coconut oil and use your fingers to rub the ingredients until they are all coated in the oil and start to clump together. Add the water and bring the dough together into a ball. It should clump and hold together but not be sticky. Add a little more water if the dough is too dry or flour if it's too sticky.

Place a sheet of parchment paper on the kitchen bench. Take half the dough, place it in the middle of the paper and cover with another sheet of parchment paper. Roll out the dough until it is the thickness of a coin (about 2 mm).

Remove the top sheet of paper and sprinkle over the sesame seeds and a little

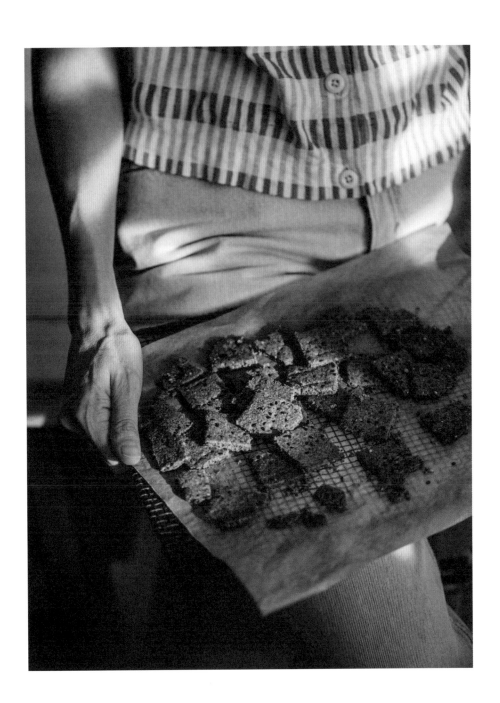

salt. Return the top sheet and roll again to press the seeds and salt into the dough. Remove the top sheet and transfer the bottom sheet, along with the dough, to a baking tray.

Score the dough into 20 or so squares and prick well with a fork. Repeat with the second batch of dough.

Bake until golden, about 15–20 minutes. Allow to cool a little before cutting along the score marks. The crackers will store well for a couple of weeks in a sealed container in a cupboard.

NOTE

Dulse is a red seaweed that is available dried as whole leaves or in flakes. This recipe calls for the latter.

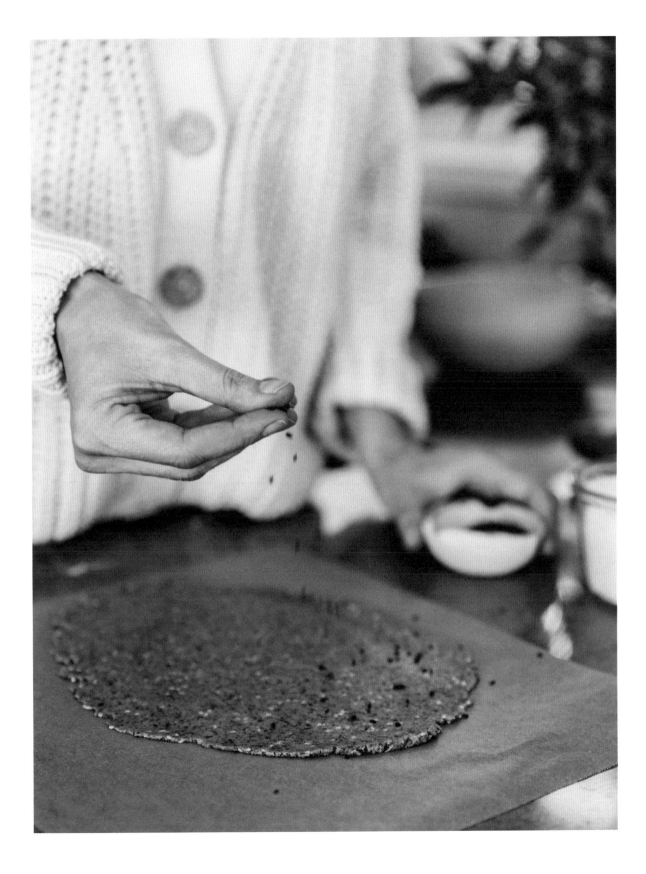

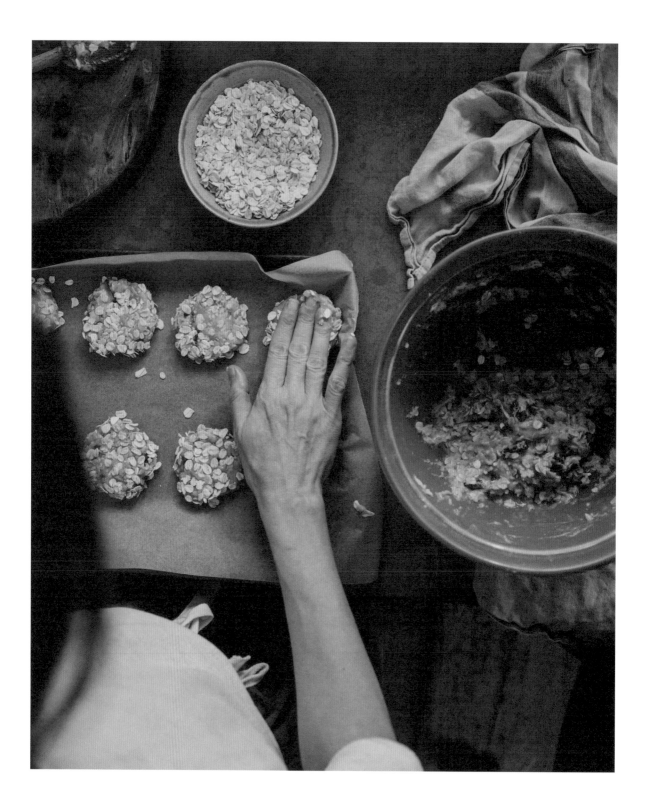

GINGERNUT BISCUITS *with* OATS *and* DRIED APRICOTS

All seasons

The measure of a good gingernut is that it remains intact after being briefly dunked into tea and is all the better for being soft and warm. These gingernuts should pass the dunk test. They are super to nibble on at the best of times, but especially if you are suffering from morning sickness, as they are more substantial than ready-made versions.

Makes *about 12 biscuits*
Time *25 minutes*

160 g (⅔ cup) extra-virgin coconut oil
90 g (¼ cup) local honey or maple syrup
185 g (1¼ cups) white wheat flour, unbleached
70 g (½ cup) whole wheat flour
75 g (⅓ cup) rolled oats, plus a handful extra in a small bowl for coating
65 g (⅓ cup) dried apricots, sulphite-free, finely chopped
2 teaspoons ground ginger
½ teaspoon bicarbonate of soda

Preheat the oven to 180°C. Line a baking tray with parchment paper.

In a small saucepan, warm the coconut oil and honey (or maple syrup) together for a few minutes. The two ingredients won't combine; however, they will become runnier and easier to mix into the dry ingredients.

Meanwhile, combine the flours, oats, apricots, ginger and bicarbonate of soda together in a large bowl. Pour in the oil and honey (or maple syrup) and stir well until no flour is visible. Scoop out a golf ball-sized amount of dough and form into a ball with your hands. Roll the ball in the extra oats to coat, then press out on the baking tray. Repeat until all the dough is used up. The biscuits can be spaced fairly close together on the baking tray as they won't spread much.

Bake until the edges have browned slightly, about 12 minutes. Leave to cool on the baking tray for 10 minutes or so before serving.

DATE, HEMP SEED *and*
ALMOND BARS

All seasons

My children love these snack bars, and I will often catch them peering hopefully into the refrigerator to see if there are any left. Sweetened only by the dates, coconut and cacao, they have no added sugar and are packed full of nourishing fats — perfect to tide you over between meals.

Makes *12 bars*
Time *20 minutes, plus 1 hour chilling*

210 g (1¼ cups) dried, pitted dates
90 g (⅓ cup) almond butter
70 g (½ cup) hemp seeds, plus extra to sprinkle on top
65 g (1 cup) desiccated coconut, unsweetened
60 ml (¼ cup) extra-virgin coconut oil
1 tablespoon ground flaxseeds (linseeds)
1 tablespoon cacao, unsweetened
25 g (¼ cup) rolled oats

Line a 20-cm square cake tin with parchment paper.

Soak the dates in boiled water until soft, about 10 minutes.

Place the almond butter, hemp seeds, coconut, coconut oil, flaxseeds and cacao in a food processor. Drain the dates, add to the other ingredients and pulse briefly until the dates are visibly chopped but the mix is still quite lumpy. Remove the bowl and blade from the processor and stir through the oats.

Transfer the mix to the prepared tin and use the back of a spoon to press it out evenly and into the corners. Sprinkle with extra hemp seeds and press gently. Refrigerate for at least 1 hour, then cut into bars. Store in an airtight container in the refrigerator.

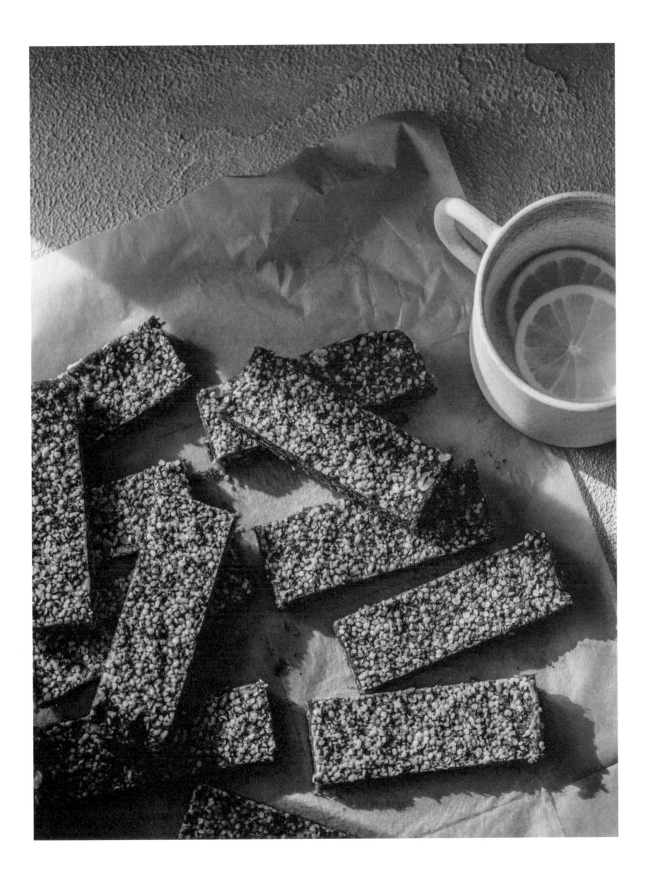

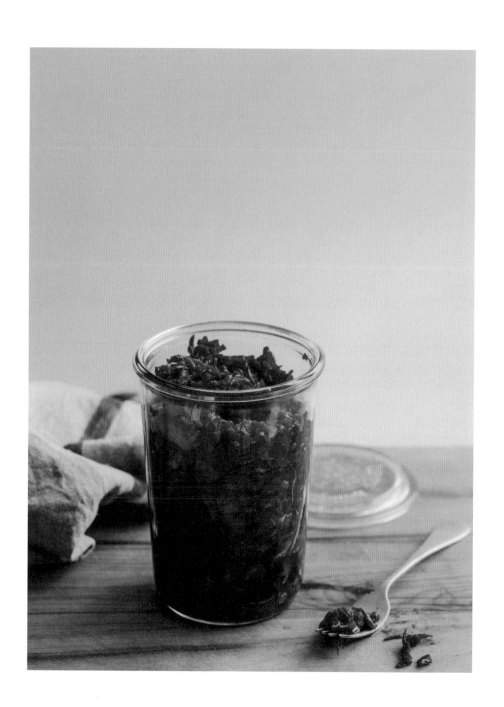

BEETROOT *and* GINGER SAUERKRAUT

All seasons
Gluten-free

This version of sauerkraut is ruby red and ever so slightly zingy from the ginger. Like other acidic seasonings (vinegar included), sauerkraut is great to have on hand to dress up a simple grain or lentil salad. Try this one with a bowl of seasoned lentils, with a little sugar, spring or finely diced red onion and citrus juice, if it's in season.

You will find mixed advice as to whether you need to sterilise your jar or crock before fermenting sauerkraut. Since I find it little effort to pop a jar in the oven while I prepare the kraut, I usually go ahead and sterilise (see page 160). Another option is to take a jar straight from the dishwasher, as the steam will have seen to any germs. We need not worry about a little bacterium here and there, since that is what we are cultivating when fermenting. Plus, the right amount of salt will keep the 'bad' bugs at bay. Choose an appropriate-sized jar for the amount of ingredients you have — you do not want too much space at the top of the ingredients for air to circulate, since fermentation happens without oxygen.

Makes *about 1 litre*
Time *15 minutes, plus around 1 week fermenting*

½ head white cabbage, cored, halved and finely shredded (keep one outer leaf to one side)
1 beetroot, topped and peeled
a large knob of ginger, peeled
salt
a sterilised jar of a suitable size

Take a large mixing bowl, place it on a set of digital scales and tare it. Add the shredded cabbage, whole peeled beetroot and ginger and weigh to work out the weight of the ingredients. Make a quick note of the weight. Remove the beetroot and ginger and set aside, as you do not want to massage these with the cabbage.

Tare the scales again. To work out how much salt you need, allow for

2 per cent of the weight of the vegetables. For example, if you have 1.5 kg of vegetables, add 30 g salt. (Alternatively, as a rule of thumb, allow 1½ teaspoons of salt per 500 g vegetables [a teaspoon of salt is about 6 g].)

Add the salt to the cabbage. Scrunch and massage the cabbage with your hands until it has softened and plenty of brine runs freely into the bowl when it is squeezed. This can take as little as 5 minutes with a small, fresh cabbage with plenty of moisture, or up to 15 minutes with a large, old cabbage that is quite dry.

Grate the beetroot and ginger into the cabbage and mix well. Transfer the kraut and ruby brine to the jar and pack down well. The brine needs to come up above the cabbage to prevent air getting to it. The jar should be around three-quarters full. Take the cabbage leaf you set aside and place this over the cabbage and push down again, so that the leaf is covered by the brine as best you can. This leaf will eventually get composted, so it is not the end of things if a little gets exposed to the air. If you have a small ceramic dish or weight, you can place this on top of the leaf to keep it weighted down under the brine.

Cover the jar with a lid and leave it to stand for a week at room temperature, then taste to see if it is to your liking. In warmer temperatures the sauerkraut will ferment faster, and in cooler temperatures it will take longer. When ready, add the top leaf to the compost and pop the sauerkraut in the refrigerator to store.

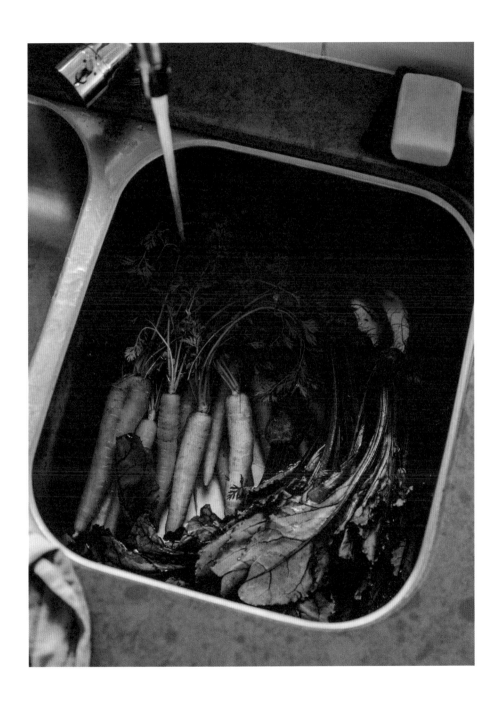

HEMP *and* DULSE GOMASHIO

All seasons

Gluten-free

Gomashio ('goma' means sesame and 'shio' means salt) is a Japanese seasoning that is used in any place that you might sprinkle salt but want a little more flavour. In this case I have added some hemp seed and dulse for nourishing fats and extra sea minerals.

Makes *about 1 cup*
Time *15 minutes*

50 g (⅓ cup) golden sesame seeds
50 g (⅓ cup) hemp seeds
1 tablespoon coarse salt
1 tablespoon dulse

Dry toast the sesame seeds in a small frying pan, tossing gently until golden and fragrant, about 3–4 minutes. Transfer to a mortar and pestle (*suribachi*) and slowly and evenly crush all the seeds to release their oils, but not completely into a powder. Transfer to a clean jar and leave to cool. When ready, add the hemp seeds, salt and dulse. Screw on the jar lid and shake to give the ingredients a good mix. Store in the refrigerator.

CULTURED PLANT YOGHURTS AND CREAM

TOASTED CASHEW YOGHURT

All seasons

Gluten-free

This yoghurt is delicious before it's cultured, so if you are short on time or if it's your preference, you can skip fermenting and enjoy it straight away.

Makes *about 2 cups*
Time *15 minutes, plus 1½ days soaking and fermenting time*

310 g (2 cups) raw unsalted cashews
310 ml (1¼ cups) chlorine-free water (see note on page 257) or milk of your choice
3–4 probiotic capsules (see note on page 257)
a sterilised jar of a suitable size

Preheat the oven to 180°C. Spread the cashew nuts on a baking tray and toast in the oven until golden, about 5 minutes.

Transfer to a high-speed blender and process until smooth, stopping to scrape down the sides if needed.

Pour in the water (or milk) and continue to blend until well combined and smooth. You can eat the yoghurt at this point or add the probiotic powder and briefly pulse again until it is incorporated.

Transfer to the jar and cover with a lid. Leave to stand in a warm place until tiny bubbles appear, about 1–2 days. Taste to check when it is to your liking and store in the refrigerator until ready to use.

COCONUT YOGHURT

All seasons

Gluten-free

Store-bought coconut yoghurt can be expensive, but it is easy enough to make at home. This recipe is for 1 x 400-ml can, but you can double the recipe if you want to make more. You might like to add a scraping of a vanilla bean pod or vanilla bean powder for extra sweetness and flavour.

Makes *400 ml*
Time *15 minutes, plus 1–2 days fermenting time*

1½ tablespoons cornflour
1 teaspoon rapadura sugar
400 ml (1½ cups and 1 tablespoon) coconut cream
1–2 probiotic capsules
a sterilised jar of a suitable size and a cook's thermometer

Place the cornflour, sugar and a dash of the liquid part of the coconut cream in a small pan and use a wooden spoon to mix them into a chalky slurry. The cornflour should be completely dissolved with no lumps. Pour in the remaining coconut cream.

Heat the coconut cream gently over a low–medium heat and stir continuously with the wooden spoon to thicken and fully dissolve the sugar.

When the coconut cream gently bubbles and starts to thicken, continue stirring for a minute and then remove from the heat. Allow the cream to cool to 40°C or lower, then stir in the powder from the probiotic capsules.

Carefully pour the thickened cream into a sterilised jar and close the lid. Wrap snugly in a folded tea towel held in place with a rubber band and leave in a warm place for a day or so. I like to use the warming plate on my coffee maker. Alternatively, you can use a yoghurt maker if you have one. Taste to see if it is to your liking, and when you are happy, store the yoghurt in the refrigerator and use within a week.

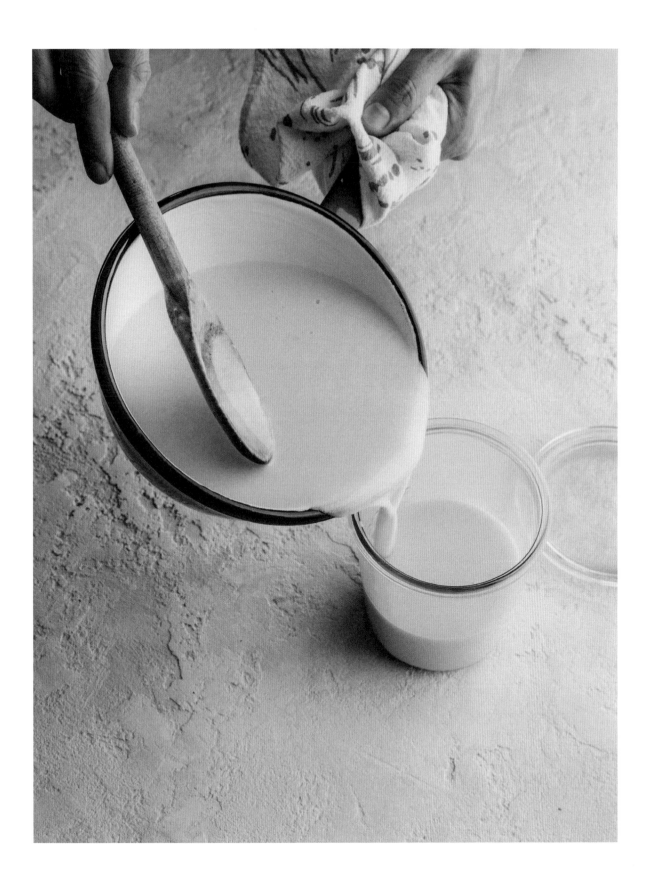

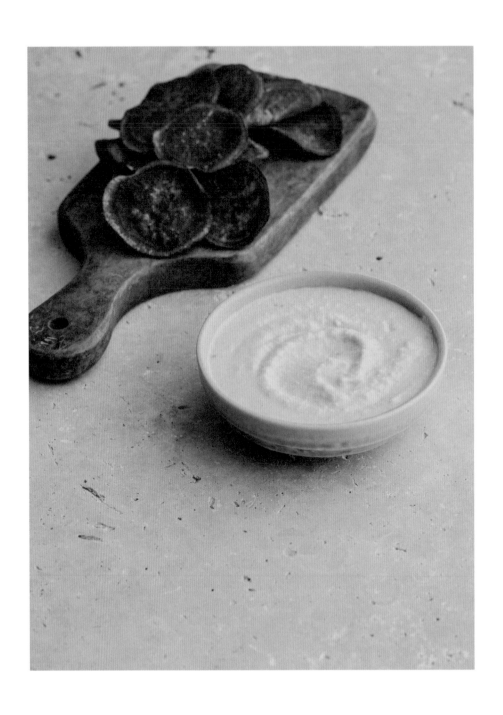

CULTURED CASHEW CREAM

All seasons

Gluten-free

Makes *1½ cups*
Time *15 minutes, plus 1½ days soaking and fermenting time*

155 g (1 cup) raw unsalted cashews
2–3 probiotic capsules (see note)
125 ml (½ cup) chlorine-free water (see note)

Cover the cashews with water and soak overnight at room temperature. This can be 'ordinary' water as it is simply to soften the nuts.

In the morning, rinse and drain the cashews and blitz with a high-speed blender until smooth. You may need to scrape down the sides a couple of times. Add the powder from the probiotic capsules and the chlorine-free water, and process again until well combined.

Transfer the cream to a clean jar, leaving a little room at the top for the cream to expand. Cover with a tea towel and hold this in place with string or an elastic band. Leave to ferment in a warm place for 24 hours, or until bubbles appear throughout, then pop a lid on the jar and refrigerate until ready to use.

NOTES

You can buy probiotic capsules from a pharmacy, some supermarkets or online. Any should work, whether shelf stable or refrigerated. The probiotic is adding bacteria that ferment the natural sugars in the nuts or grains and give that tangy flavour that you find in yoghurt and other cultured foods. As an alternative to capsules, you could use a tablespoon of yoghurt (dairy or plant-based) as your probiotic source, since these products have already been combined with probiotics by the producer. If you plan to make more cultured cream or yoghurt after your first batch, you can reserve some and use this as your starter next time.

Municipal tap water usually contains chlorine, chloramine and fluoride which can inhibit fermentation. There are three options to remove these inhibitors. Working from fast to slow: 1. Filter the water, 2. Boil the water (allow to cool before using), or 3. Stand the water in an uncovered bowl overnight.

Chapter 8

THE SCIENCE OF NUTRITION

Nutrition science should not be mistaken for the study of individual nutrients, but rather the lessons taught by their collective social lives — the context that affects their presence and behaviour, how they relate with each, and the patterns that emerge as a consequence. Nutrition science explores all of this and, in doing so, is far more complex than we are sometimes led to believe. That is why this chapter is towards the end of this book; that, and the notion that though we ought not need knowledge of nutrients to eat well, taught holistically and with humility, nutrition science offers an alternative way of appreciating the interconnectedness of it all.

Knowing Food Differently

Nutrients are compounds or elements that the body makes use of to support life. As the human body evolved over many millions of years, it came upon an uncountable assortment of nutrients, which were provided by the enormous diversity of plants and animals in the many places our forebears lived. However, even within that mix, there exists some order — nutrients that the body has come to find function for, and in a way expects, from our foodways.

Some nutrients are generally eaten in relatively large amounts. These are called *macronutrients* and include fats, proteins and carbohydrates. They make up the bulk of food and are measured in grams. Macronutrients can be reduced further into even smaller parts. For example, there are 20 amino acids that join together in many different ways to form proteins. Other nutrients are needed in somewhat smaller amounts and are measured in units of one thousandth of a gram (milligram — mg) or one millionth of a gram (microgram — μg). These are known as *micronutrients* and include compounds called vitamins and certain elements, usually referred to as minerals.

The body can make some nutrients, whereas others must come from food and, in one specific case, sunshine. There can be aspects of interchangeability, where a function in the body can be fulfilled by more than one nutrient. For example, energy can be produced by metabolising fats, proteins or carbohydrates. However, in most cases, functions can only be performed by specific nutrients. In these instances, and when the nutrient cannot be made by the body, they are called essential nutrients.

By studying the effects of differing amounts of nutrients in foodways and levels in the body, scientists have suggested prescriptions that when met seem to promote proper body functioning. These are known as *nutritional requirements*. Requirements are set on a population basis, meaning they are levels that are considered to provide enough for almost everyone. Some people may need much less, and some more — they are approximations.

Nutritional requirements change over the course of life. The body needs higher intakes of some nutrients during seasons when it is growing, such as in infancy, childhood, adolescence, pregnancy and during breastfeeding. At times, the body can adapt its metabolism of nutrients to go some way towards meeting needs in circumstances of higher demand or if intakes are low. Nutritional requirements are not set in stone — they are changeable.

Foods are changeable as well. Nutrition labels give an illusion that foods are standardised packages of a handful of nutrients. But they are not. Foods are an embodiment of the ecology in which they were grown. A chicken that scrubs around in dirt, picking out insects, will produce eggs that are different (nutritionally speaking) to the eggs of a chicken confined to a cage, fed a concoction of synthetic chemicals and antibiotics. Far from uniformity, foods and the components from which they are made are diverse. They contain a rich array of bioactive compounds that interact *with each other and the body* in complex ways — which can be easy to lose sight of when looking at single nutrients and prescriptive nutritional requirements.

The discovery of nutrients, and the beginnings of nutrition as a science, can be traced back to a time when the body was viewed like a mechanical machine. For decades, scientists thought that the key to understanding how the machine worked was by investigating its component parts and how they fitted together. While there is nothing wrong with exploring the components from which living beings are made, this reductive view of life tells only part of a story.

The structures from which life is made cannot tell us of their *properties* — how they behave in context. Properties are emergent. They are not found at the level of a part but at the level of the whole system. The saying 'the whole is more than the sum of its parts' leans into this holistic view. We appreciate now that the body is not a machine. It is a complex, interconnected system made of webs of relationships that braid everything together. No nutrient works on its own, independent of others, and without a biological system to interact with.

Macronutrients

Fats

Fats perform three main functions in the body. The first is energy-giving — to provide the fuel for growth, movement and simply *being*. The second is metabolic — to provide the materials needed to make compounds that resolve all manner of inflammation and oxidative damage. The third is structural — to create the fabric of cell membranes.[172] Any dietary fat that is eaten beyond what is used for these functions is stored for later.

It is not uncommon for attention to be directed to the effects of stored fats on the body, creating a weight-centric view of health. But not only can a focus on weight be damaging to our view of our bodies and relationship with food, but it can also mean losing sight of the absolute centrality of dietary fats in keeping us well.

Of the wide array of fats that exist in food, there are only two that are considered essential — *alpha-linolenic acid* (ALA) and *linoleic acid* (LA), both of which come from plants. These essential fats are more commonly referred to by their chemical structure — omega-3 and omega-6.[10] Both are 'parents' that can produce 'families' of very long chain fats in the body; ALA

---

10   For clarity, the numbers 3 and 6 simply relate to the position of a double bond in a carbon chain counting backwards from one end; where omega, being the last letter of the Greek alphabet, is the final point. Though seemingly a subtle difference, the position of the double bond in the carbon chain significantly affects the structure, function and stability of the fat.

produces the omega-3 family which includes *eicosapentaenoic acid* (EPA) and *docosahexaenoic acid* (DHA), and LA produces the omega-6 family which includes *arachidonic acid* (AA).

The very long chain omega-3 DHA is notable because it is the main component of the brain cells of all animals. The presence of DHA in the brains of animals is thought to stretch as far back as 600 million years, in other words, the entirety of animal evolution.[173] This is *extreme conservation* and shows that DHA is irreplaceable — nothing has come along since that could more effectively perform the jobs DHA does.[174, 175] What separates human brains from those of other animals is not their structure or chemistry, but simply their size. And big brains need a ready supply of DHA to function well.

While humans *can* make very long chain omega-3s from shorter chain omega-3s (and this is why DHA is not classed as essential), our capacity to do so is limited. What is more, high intakes of omega-6s impair the metabolism of very long chain omega-3s, because they make use of the same enzyme. This interaction between omega-3s and omega-6s would not have mattered in the context of ancient times. Ancestral foodways would have been rich in both shorter and very long chain omega-3s. However, modern diets usually contain low amounts of omega-3s and high amounts of omega-6s. The ratio can be around 1:20, which contrasts to a ratio in ancestral foodways of 1:2.[176] A number of changes have contributed to this swing:

> 1. *From leaves to seeds*: with a few exceptions, omega-3s are generally more concentrated in leaves and omega-6s in seeds. Nowadays, not only do people eat considerably fewer leaves than in ancient times, but they also eat markedly more seeds as grains (grains are the seeds of grasses) and seed oils (e.g. palm oil, cottonseed oil, rapeseed/canola oil). As human foodways have transitioned over the millennia, so too have the diets of the animals that are eaten. Industrial animal

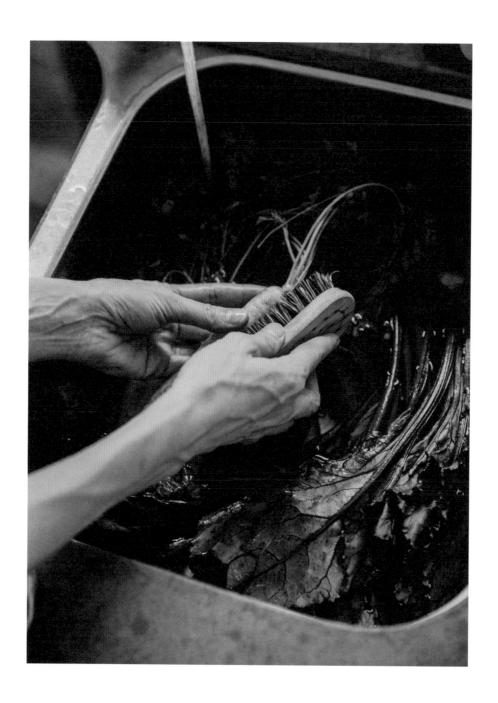

production practices have shifted the diets of farm animals away from leaves (and in the case of poultry, insects) to seeds (grains and legumes). As with humans, this transition has lowered the omega-3 and raised the omega-6 content of meat, milk and eggs.

2. *From water to land*: ancestral foodways would have contained plentiful amounts of long chain omega-3s from foods found near fresh water sources, such as lakes, rivers and streams.[177] Analysed bone specimens from the mid-upper Paleolithic period show that between 10 and 50 per cent of the diet of early modern humans came from fish, shellfish, turtles/tortoises and water fowl.[178] The meat from land animals contains fewer long chain omega-3s.

3. *From whole to part*: lastly, quite unlike the modern experience of trimming fats from meat and choosing to eat only lean cuts, our ancestors would have eaten all parts of the animal including their fatty tissue and brains, which would have provided plentiful omega-3s.

Foods that are rich in essential fats are of great value in the pre-conceptual period — high intakes improve fertility in both sexes.[179] In women, fats are the basis for many hormones involved in the menstrual cycle and a high intake of omega-3 DHA, in particular, is associated with a reduced risk of anovulation.[180] In men, the sperm and testes contain much more omega-3 DHA than other parts of the body (apart from the brain and eyes).[181] In the sperm tail, fats provide the fluidity, flexibility and energy needed to achieve fertilisation. Incidentally, this is also why fish contain high levels of omega-3 DHA, to allow for the same sort of movement.[182, 183] Given sperm are regularly replenished, it is important that men routinely get good amounts of essential fats from their foodways. Essential fats are also key in pregnancy, breastfeeding and the first couple of years of life, because this is when the majority of human brain development takes place.

While oily fish are the richest sources of very long chain omega-3s, even at current levels of fish consumption, fisheries cannot sustainably keep pace with demand. There are few alternative food sources of very long chain omega-3s. Pastured chicken and eggs may provide small amounts if eaten regularly. If little or no fish is eaten, getting plenty of plant foods that are rich in omega-3 ALA is key. But it is equally important to think about choosing culinary oils that are low in omega-6s and using them judiciously, as these can be major contributors to the high omega-6 to omega-3 ratio seen in modern times.

TYPICAL DAILY OMEGA-3 NEEDS

Pre-pregnancy — 0.8 g ALA
Pregnancy — 1.0 g ALA
Breastfeeding — 1.2 g ALA

NOTABLE SOURCES OF OMEGA-3

Plants — dark leafy greens, walnuts, some seeds (and their oils) including chia, flax (linseeds) and hemp seeds
Animals — fish (especially oily), meat (especially pasture-raised), eggs (especially free range)
Low omega-6 oils — olive oil, coconut oil, rapeseed oil, almond oil

NOTABLE SOURCES OF OMEGA-6

Plants — most seeds (and their oils) including pumpkin, sesame and sunflower, grains
Animals — animal fats are a mixture of fats including omega-6. Animals that are grazed have less omega-6 and more omega-3 than those that are grain fed.[184]

Protein

All enzymes and many hormones and immune factors are proteins, making protein fundamental for metabolism. Proteins also have a structural role, for example in muscles, skin, bones and connective tissue, meaning that protein requirements are higher during times of growth, as in pregnancy and breastfeeding. Proteins are made from base compounds called amino acids. Ordinarily, nine amino acids are classed as essential and the remaining eleven are non-essential. However, towards the end of pregnancy, it seems the body is unable to make sufficient glycine to meet the higher demands, and it too can be considered essential at this time.[185]

Plant foods are often perceived as being substandard when it comes to protein. The roots of this view lie in some clumsy wording that initially grouped protein sources according to their essential amino acid content as either complete or incomplete. Plant foods were generally classed as being incomplete — implying that they were missing one or more essential amino acids. However, this is not the case — we know now that all plant foods contain all 20 amino acids, including the nine essential amino acids. This negative perception of plant sources of protein was stirred by reductive rather than holistic thinking.

While tests of single foods do show that plant foods are often lower than animal foods in some essential amino acids, this does not matter when a variety of plant foods are eaten over the course of a day. This is true even of vegan foodways that include no animal protein sources at all, as well as during times of higher protein needs, for example in pregnancy, infancy and childhood. Protein intakes in upper income countries are usually much higher than requirements.

TYPICAL DAILY PROTEIN NEEDS

Pre-pregnancy — 46 g
Pregnancy — 60 g
Breastfeeding — 67 g

> *Plants — whole grains, pulses, nuts, seeds*
> *Animals — meat, fish, eggs, milk and other dairy products*

Carbohydrates

Just as fats are made from the building blocks of fatty acids and proteins are made from amino acids, carbohydrates have building blocks too — sugars. The body can't digest all carbohydrates, as it lacks the necessary enzymes to do so. But for those that it can, enzymes split carbohydrate chains down to sugars before absorbing them. Digestible carbohydrates are similar to other macronutrients in that they provide energy, however, unlike proteins and fats, energy provision is their only function. Given that other macronutrients may also provide energy, there are no nutritional requirements for carbohydrates in the same way there are for essential fats and proteins.

Only a small amount of glucose (about 50 grams) is actually needed for brain function, and this is easily provided for in varied foodways. However, whole plant foods are also rich in 'non-digestible' carbohydrates, such as cellulose. Once eaten, this fibre passes through the gut and into the large intestine where it is fermented by microbiota to produce beneficial compounds that are then absorbed. And so, unlike digestible carbohydrates, there is a recommended amount of fibrous carbohydrates to promote gut health.

Despite there being no substantial need for digestible carbohydrates, history tells us that there is no reason to believe that carbohydrate-containing foods cannot be included as part of nourishing foodways. It is the case that carbohydrate-rich grains only became a staple food in many societies after the agricultural revolution. However, even before then, foods containing carbohydrates would have been a common feature of ancestral foodways. Carbohydrate food sources would have included roots and tubers, as well as nuts, seeds, fruit, honey and the inner bark of some trees, such as maple and birch.[186] Though animal foods may well have been revered in the same way they are by many people today, the energy used to hunt for animals would have been far more than that used collecting tubers and such.[187] Scientists think it likely that roots and tubers would have been particularly important in the foodways of early humans.

With the transition to agrarian foodways, humans began eating more and more grains in place of wild plant foods. Eventually with industrialisation, large amounts of highly refined grains and added sugars have found their way into foodways, but bodies have not evolved at an equal pace to deal with these effectively. It is these differences that may account for the adverse health effects of modern carbohydrate-containing products, rather than it being a consequence of the carbohydrates per se. Enjoying minimally processed foods like whole grains and pulses and including plenty of vegetables draws us back more closely to nourishing ancestral foodways and also ensures we get plenty of fibre (see also Bringing Balance, page 95).

TYPICAL DAILY FIBRE NEEDS

Pre-pregnancy — 25 g
Pregnancy — 28 g
Breastfeeding — 30 g

NOTABLE SOURCES OF FIBRE

Plants — whole grains, pulses, nuts and seeds, vegetables and fruit

Micronutrients

Vitamin A

For almost 3 billion years, long before the evolution of early modern humans, vitamin A has been essential for enabling life (microorganisms, plants and animals) to absorb sunlight and allowing vision (or the equivalent of vision), as well as in part controlling the body clock.[188]

Vitamin A was the first vitamin to be identified and is not one but a large group of similar compounds. The scientific name for vitamin A is retinol, which comes from the word *retina*, because vitamin A is essential for eyesight. Humans have evolved many other uses for vitamin A, including creating the body plan by controlling cell growth and differentiation from the embryo stage right through into adulthood. Vitamin A is also a protective antioxidant and supports the immune system.

Broadly speaking, there are two types of vitamin A — retinol, which is found in animal foods, and carotenes. Carotenes are mostly found in colourful vegetables and fruit, but they are also found in some fish and shellfish — they are what give wild salmon its pink colour (farmed fish are given carotene supplements to mimic this effect). Carotenes are sometimes called *pro-vitamin A* as the body converts them to retinol, as and when needed.

More than 600 carotenes have been identified but only a handful are routinely consumed, the most common one being beta-carotene. You may be familiar with the adage of eating carrots to help you see in the dark and this is where that comes from. Carrots are rich in beta-carotene, which your body converts to vitamin A and uses to maintain good vision.

Vitamin A plays many roles in reproduction for both sexes. For men, it is crucial for making sperm, and in women, it is used throughout pregnancy, especially in the development of the placenta. Deficiency of vitamin A has been shown to cause infertility or reduce the chance of successfully conceiving. Notably in men, vitamin A deficiency halts the production of sperm and testosterone. On the other hand, high intakes of vitamin A in its retinol form have been shown to be teratogenic and toxic to the developing embryo (see also Caretaking, page 116). This is not the case for carotenes, where the only known side effect of getting too much is that your skin may glow a little yellow–orange.

TYPICAL DAILY VITAMIN A NEEDS

Pre-pregnancy — 700 µg
Pregnancy — 800 µg
Breastfeeding — 1100 µg
Maximum at any adult life stage — 3000 µg

> *Plants — dark leafy greens, colourful fruit and*
> *vegetables (especially orange coloured)*
> *Animals — fish (especially wild and oily), liver,* kidney, cod*
> *liver oil,* milk (especially pasture raised), other dairy products,*
> *e.g. yoghurt, butter, and eggs (especially free range)*
> **High intakes of vitamin A can be teratogenic and should be*
> *avoided during pregnancy. See also Caretaking, page 116.*

Vitamin B complex

There are eight vitamins that make up the B group, which is confusing as there is a B9 and a B12. This group is sometimes referred to together as the B complex because their roles are closely interwoven with each other. The B complex includes B1 (thiamin), B2 (riboflavin), B3 (niacin), B5 (pantothenic acid), B6 (pyridoxine), B7 (biotin), B9 (folate) and B12 (cobalamin). Attention is given here to those B vitamins that are especially relevant in early motherhood, either due to elevated requirements or challenges with meeting needs.

FOLATE

Folate is also known as vitamin B9, and is not actually one vitamin, but a group of similar compounds called vitamers. Like in almost all other living organisms, folate is essential for metabolism and is involved in creating nucleotides, which are the building blocks of DNA. Low folate levels or deficiency can develop when dietary intake is inadequate, but also with poor absorption when requirements are increased, such as during pregnancy and breastfeeding, or with certain genetic mutations. Folate levels can also be compromised when intakes of other vitamins in the B complex are low, specifically, vitamins B6, B12 and B2 (riboflavin), as these are all needed for folate metabolism.

The word folate comes from the Latin word *folium*, meaning foliage or leaf, because leafy greens are an excellent source of this essential nutrient. For most of human history, our ancestors would have foraged on an abundance of wild leafy greens, and other plants, including fruit, making their foodways rich in folate. Consequently, humans are biologically attuned to obtaining considerable amounts of this nutrient from food. Unfortunately, modern foodways are often notably lacking in folate.

TYPICAL DAILY FOLATE NEEDS

Pre-pregnancy — 400 µg, plus supplement 400 ug/d at least 4 weeks before conception
Pregnancy — 600 µg, plus supplement 400 ug/d for first 12 weeks
Breastfeeding — 500 µg
NB Folate supplements are recommended before and in early pregnancy. See also Folate, pages 298 and 301.

NOTABLE SOURCES OF FOLATE

Plants — raw or lightly cooked dark leafy greens, beans, peanuts, sunflower seeds, fruit, whole grains
Animals — eggs, liver,* milk (fresh only, not long life)
* There are some considerations around eating liver in pregnancy. See also Caretaking, page 116.

VITAMIN B12

Vitamin B12 performs many important functions in the body, including cell growth and development. One of the signs of B12 deficiency is enlarged red blood cells and a smaller than normal amount, called megaloblastic anaemia. This means that the blood cells are not as effective at their job in carrying oxygen around the body. Vitamin B12 also supports in creating the protective covering that wraps around nerves, and deficiency can lead to irreversible nerve damage. This has been found in babies born to mothers with inadequate B12 intakes during pregnancy.

Vitamin B12 is unique amongst all micronutrients in that it is only made by some microbial species, namely certain bacteria and similar primitive microorganisms, called archaea.[189] Some of these B12-producing microbes live in our guts, however, they are only found in our large intestine. This is an unfortunate quirk of physiology because we can only absorb B12 from our small intestine, which comes first. Because of this oddity and the fact that B12 is essential for survival, B12 must come from foods.

There are various ways animals can get their B12. Herbivores don't have the same quirk of biology as humans do and can absorb B12 from the microbes in their guts. From there, animals store it in their tissues, so eating this meat would have been the main way our ancestors would have met their B12 needs (though it is possible they also got small amounts of B12 from leading less hygienic lifestyles). Humans are able to store B12 and the amounts needed are relatively low compared with other nutrients. However, if animal meat or other foods from animals are not eaten on a daily basis, a B12 supplement may be needed (see also Supplements for Plant-based Eating, page 293).

TYPICAL DAILY B12 NEEDS

Pre-pregnancy — 2.4 mg
Pregnancy — 2.6 mg
Breastfeeding — 2.8 mg

NOTABLE SOURCES OF VITAMIN B12

Plants — none
Animals
   Egg (1 medium) — 0.6 mg
   Cow's milk (100 ml) — 0.6 mg
   Yoghurt (150 g) — 0.8 mg
   Hard cheese (25 g) — 0.4 mg
   Fish (100 g, cooked) — 3.1 mg
   Chicken (100 g, cooked) — 0.5 mg
   Beef (100 g, cooked) — 2.0 mg
Nutritional yeast (7 g/2 tablespoons) — 0.5 mg

NB These figures are provided as a guide. Actual levels may vary.

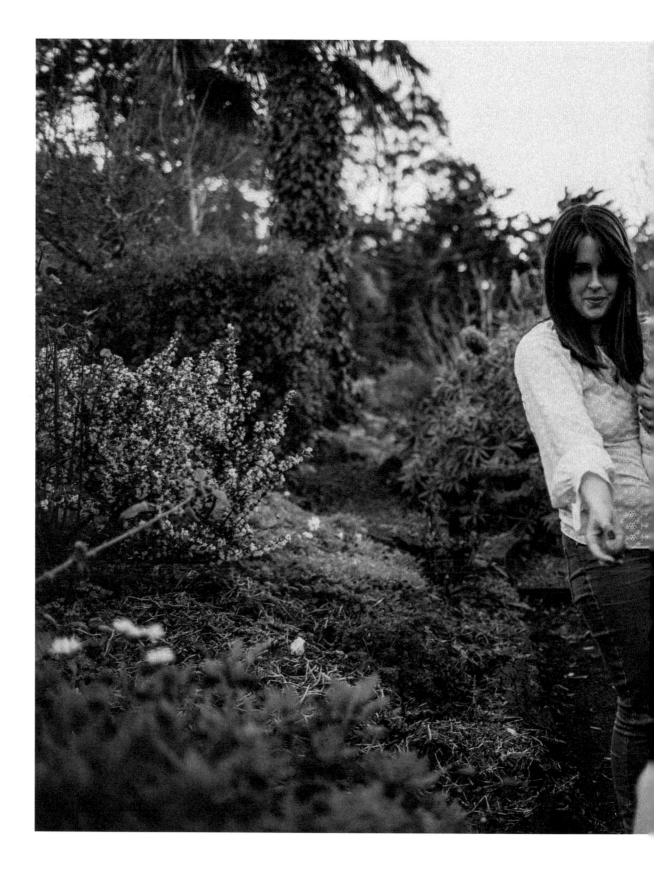

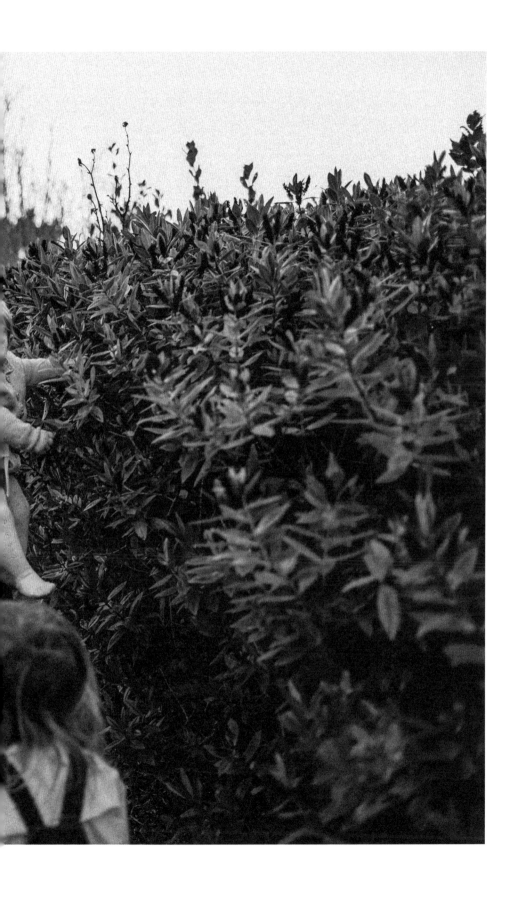

Vitamin C

Vitamin C is an antioxidant that has many functions, including protecting cells from damage, supporting the immune system, and helping with the absorption of iron from foods when eaten at the same time. Some 30–40 million years ago, a chance mutation switched off the gene that enabled the human body to make vitamin C.[190] The remnant of this gene is still present in our DNA, but inactive. Our primate relatives also cannot make vitamin C, but most other mammals can.

The fact that our ancestors could not make vitamin C, even though it is essential, means that they would have had ready access to vitamin C-rich foods. Vitamin C is found in high amounts in fresh fruit, particularly berries and citrus, and many vegetables. Ancestral foodways may have also included good amounts of vitamin C from raw organ meats.

TYPICAL DAILY VITAMIN C NEEDS

Pre-pregnancy — 45 mg
Pregnancy — 60 mg
Breastfeeding — 85 mg

NOTABLE SOURCES OF VITAMIN C

Plants — fruit (especially citrus, berries, kiwis), vegetables, fresh peas, potato family (especially capsicum (peppers)), broccoli
Animals — liver*
* There are some considerations around eating liver in pregnancy. See also Caretaking, page 116.

Vitamin D

Vitamin D is usually known for its role in calcium and phosphorus metabolism and its essentiality for healthy bones. Inadequate vitamin D can lead to rickets. However, low vitamin D levels have also been linked to several chronic conditions including autoimmune diseases and cancer, and it is understood to be vital for fertility.[191] Vitamin D is quite different to the other micronutrients because it is a hormone rather than a nutrient per se. And while some foods contain small amounts, vitamin D is mainly produced through the action of sunlight on skin.

Humans evolved in equatorial Africa where they spent most of their time outdoors, wearing little if any clothing. This meant that our ancestors would have maintained year-round high levels of vitamin D, even with the natural sunscreen effects of darker skin.[192] As generations of people moved away from the equator and dispersed further north, where there are fewer days per year when vitamin D can be produced, scientists have theorised that some groups evolved lighter skin colour (with less sun-blocking pigment) to help the production of vitamin D at higher latitudes.[193] In all populations that have been studied, females have lighter skin than males, which may enable more effective vitamin D production to support reproductive health.[194]

How much vitamin D you can make is highly dependent on where you are in the world and the amount of UVB sunlight that reaches your skin. Globally, vitamin D deficiency is highly prevalent and probably because of a mismatch between genes and environment. Factors such as clothing, time outdoors and skin colour make a difference — more body covering, less time outdoors and darker skin can all contribute to a reduced amount of vitamin D production. Those at risk of vitamin D deficiency may need a supplement (see also Vitamin D, page 292).

TYPICAL DAILY VITAMIN D NEEDS

Pre-pregnancy — 5 mg
Pregnancy — 5 mg
Breastfeeding — 5 mg

NOTABLE SOURCES OF VITAMIN D

Sunshine
Plants — *mushrooms exposed to UV light*
Animals — *oily fish, eggs (c. 2.5 mg per egg)*

Vitamin E

A century ago, scientists were investigating milk as a potential 'perfect food' — something that could meet all nutritional needs on its own (remembering the reductive approach to nutrition in its heyday). They found that while rats could initially grow well on only milk, they were unable to reproduce[11].[(195)] Subsequent experiments found that wheat germ oil contained something, initially termed 'Factor X', that was needed for fertility. With vitamins A, B, C and D already discovered by this point, Factor X was named vitamin E and was given the scientific term *tocopherol*, which comes from the ancient Greek words *tokos* meaning childbirth and *phero* meaning to bring forth. Eight forms of vitamin E have since been identified.

Although not its only function, Vitamin E is a powerful antioxidant — it works to neutralise reactive compounds called oxidants and free radicals. This is a particularly important job to protect cell membranes (rich in polyunsaturated fats) from oxidative damage. High levels of oxidation may reduce fertility and adversely affect embryonic development.

Polyunsaturated fats include several double bonds in their chemical structure, which makes them very susceptible to damage. When oils are exposed to air for too long, they become rancid in taste and smell. This is because the polyunsaturated fats break down. A similar damaging oxidative process would happen in plants and animals if there wasn't a way of preventing this, which is where vitamin E comes in as an antioxidant. Plants make protective vitamin E and mainly keep this together with the polyunsaturated fats in their energy stores, such as in nuts, seeds, whole grains.

A large proportion of the global population (across all income groups) have intakes and body levels of vitamin E that fall short of requirements. This is best remedied by eating more whole plant foods, including vegetables, and small amounts of nuts and seeds.

---

11   We now know that milk does contain vitamin E in the butterfat and there were probably some discrepancies in these early experiments where the amount of butterfat was not well controlled.

> *Pre-pregnancy — 7 mg*
> *Pregnancy — 7 mg*
> *Breastfeeding — 11 mg*

NOTABLE SOURCES OF VITAMIN E

> *Plants — leafy greens, nuts, seeds, whole grains*
> *Animals — butter (especially grass fed), fatty meat*

Calcium

Calcium is the most abundant mineral in the body. It has many roles, including supporting the transmission of nerve impulses and the release of hormones. The majority of calcium, however, is found in teeth and bones where it plays a strengthening role. The body's need for calcium is particularly high during periods when bones are forming, such as in infancy, childhood and adolescence. The second half of pregnancy and breastfeeding are other notable times when there is greater need. However, there are several changes to calcium metabolism in the peripartum period, which mean there is no call for extra calcium from food at these times. Adaptations include more efficient recycling of calcium in the body and enhanced absorption from the digestive tract.[196]

While calcium is essential for healthy bones, it is not the only nutrient that is involved in skeletal health. Dietary patterns that are low in fruit and vegetables, high in meat, salt and certain additives, promote body acidity, which prompts the body to release neutralising calcium from the bones.[197] Vitamin D also works closely with calcium to support bone health. Prior to the agricultural revolution, the calcium in ancestral foodways would have almost entirely come from wild plant foods.[198]

TYPICAL DAILY CALCIUM NEEDS

> *Pre-pregnancy — 1000 mg*
> *Pregnancy — 1000 mg*
> *Breastfeeding — 1000 mg*

> *Plants — green leafy vegetables (excluding spinach),*
> *beans, nuts, seeds, dried fruit, calcium-set tofu*
> *Animals — dairy products (including milk, cheese,*
> *yoghurt), fish (especially with soft bones), seafood*

Iodine

The primary use of iodine is in the production of thyroid hormones that control the speed of metabolism. Iodine is also involved in the development of the brain and nervous system, making it key during pregnancy and breastfeeding. Insufficient iodine in the peripartum period can impair the physical and cognitive development of babies and children.[199]

While iodine is only needed in very small amounts, deficiency is common throughout the world. The reason why is unclear, as deficiency is not limited to those countries where people have access to fewer iodine-rich foods.[200] One theory is that the transition of foodways to include more grains and other plant foods that contain iodine blockers (goitrogens) may have simultaneously increased the demand for thyroid hormones (which are important for carbohydrate metabolism). In other words, modern iodine requirements could be higher than what our ancestors needed.[201–203]

In nature, iodine is scarce on land, as most of it has long been washed away into the sea. As a result, key natural food sources of iodine are those that are marine-based, such as fish, shellfish and sea vegetables. If you live close to coastal seaweed beds, it has even been suggested that you can inhale significant amounts of iodine from the sea air.[204] Although, it's probably best not to rely on this to meet needs!

On land, the thyroid glands of animals contain the largest known amounts of iodine, but these don't feature much on modern menus. Cows raised on feed rather than pasture will produce meat and milk that is higher in iodine because their feed is supplemented with it. Iodine is also used in the sterilisers that clean the equipment used for milking, making dairy foods adventitiously good sources. Otherwise, the iodine content of land-based plants and other animals is generally low.

Due to concerns around iodine deficiency, some countries, including Australia and New Zealand, have laws that require the salt used in bread to be iodised. However, many others do not, including the US and much of Europe. Sea salt contains almost no iodine, compared to iodised salt with 44 µg/1 g. If fish, seafood and/or dairy are not eaten regularly, an iodine supplement may be needed (see also Supplements for Plant-based Eating, page 293).

TYPICAL DAILY IODINE NEEDS

Pre-pregnancy — 150 µg
Pregnancy — 250 µg
Breastfeeding — 250 µg

NOTABLE SOURCES OF IODINE

Plants — sea vegetables (brown > red > green)*, iodine-fortified plant milks
Animals
Egg (1 medium) 19 mg
Cow's milk (100 ml) 23 mg
Yoghurt (150 g) 38 mg
Hard cheese (25 g) 6 mg
Fish (100 g, cooked) 29 mg
*See notes on sea vegetables in pregnancy (Foods from Plants, page 45).

Iron

Most of the body's iron is found in red blood cells, where it helps to transport oxygen around the body. Iron also plays a key role in energy production, protein building and immunity. Globally, iron deficiency is the most common cause of anaemia and affects almost a quarter of the world's population. Iron deficiency anaemia can lead to fertility issues in both men and women, including ovulatory infertility. In upper income countries, low intakes are usually the main cause of low iron levels.

There are two different forms of iron in foods, *haem* and *non-haem*. Both of these are found in animal foods, but plant foods only contain the latter. Haem iron is much better absorbed than non-haem iron, and there are also compounds in some plant foods that cling to minerals including iron, zinc, calcium and manganese, preventing their absorption. Vitamin C enhances plant-based iron absorption, so eating fruit and vegetables with meals helps, even if they contain little iron in their own right.

TYPICAL DAILY IRON NEEDS

Pre-pregnancy — 18 mg
Pregnancy — 27 mg
Breastfeeding — 9 mg

NOTABLE SOURCES OF IRON

Plants — pulses, nuts, dried fruit (e.g. dates, figs), leafy greens, herbs (if eaten in good amounts), tofu, whole grains
Animals — meat, fish, seafood

Selenium

Selenium is an antioxidant mineral that is important for the immune system and the production of thyroid hormones. Low selenium levels have been linked to adverse pregnancy outcomes including preeclampsia, gestational diabetes, and preterm birth.[205] In men, selenium is essential for healthy sperm and fertility. Selenium is a key component of several proteins that are involved in the normal growth and functioning of sperm, including specifically in the midsection of the tail.[206] Part of selenium's beneficial role also relates to its antioxidant function, as sperm are very susceptible to oxidative damage. Some (but not all) studies have found that supplementation with selenium improves sperm quality.[207, 208] Selenium is also needed to make testosterone.

Selenium enters the food web through plants, but unlike in humans, it is not essential for plant survival and levels in plant foods are generally

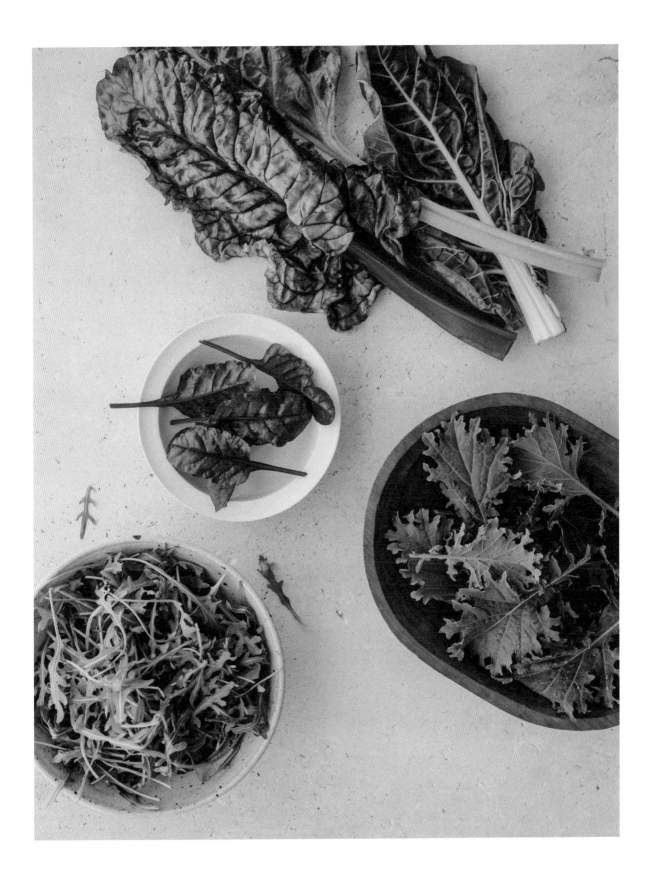

low. What is more, the amount of selenium in plants is dependent on the selenium content of the soil in which they are grown, and dietary intakes vary geographically. Areas with low soil selenium contents include the UK, New Zealand, Australia, and parts of Europe. Soils in some areas of China, the US, Canada and India are rich in selenium, whereas other areas are low.[209] It can be difficult to know whether selenium intakes are an issue because it depends a lot on where food comes from.

TYPICAL DAILY SELENIUM NEEDS

> *Pre-pregnancy — 60 mg*
> *Pregnancy — 65 mg*
> *Breastfeeding — 75 mg*
> *Men — 70 mg*

NOTABLE SOURCES OF SELENIUM

> *Plants — Brazil nuts, cashew nuts, whole grains grown in*
> *selenium-replete soils (e.g. US but not European), sesame seeds*
> *Animals — organ meats (especially liver* and*
> *kidney), fish,[12] shellfish, red meat, eggs*
> ** There are some considerations around eating liver*
> *in pregnancy. See also Caretaking, page 116.*

Zinc

Zinc is a mineral that is found in every cell in the body. It performs a wide range of functions, including speeding up many of the enzymes that run metabolism and supporting DNA expression. In relation to fertility and pregnancy, zinc is essential for hormonal rhythms, embryo formation and development, and inadequate intakes can affect growth and development and increase the risk of malformations, including neural tube defects.

---

12   In fish and seafood, selenium combines with mercury or methylmercury (both damaging to sperm) and renders these unavailable. However, in doing so, the bioavailability of selenium is also reduced.

Beyond the peripartum period, zinc is so widely used by the body that deficiency can cause many issues, for example, impaired healing after injury, dermatitis and neurological disorders.[210]

Zinc is found in plant and animal foods that are high in protein. There are plentiful sources of zinc, however, some plant foods contain compounds called phytates that can reduce zinc absorption (see also Anti-nutrients, below). Alcohol also affects zinc metabolism. Indeed, many of the effects of foetal alcohol syndrome can be directly attributed to zinc deficiency rather than the effects of alcohol per se.[211] When little or no animal foods are eaten, it is important to be mindful of food practices that reduce phytates to promote mineral absorption, including zinc (see also Anti-nutrients, below).

TYPICAL DAILY ZINC NEEDS

Pre-pregnancy — 8 mg
Pregnancy — 11 mg
Breastfeeding — 12 mg

NOTABLE SOURCES OF ZINC

Plants — pulses, nuts (especially toasted), seeds, whole grains
Animals — meat, fish, seafood, eggs

Anti-nutrients

There are various compounds in plant foods that have been pinpointed as possible factors that can block or reduce the absorption of some minerals. These include oxalates, phytates, tannins and goitrogens. Their discovery has led some to question the ability of foodways based mostly or entirely on plants to meet nutritional requirements. However, foods are not eaten in isolation and many of these compounds are reduced through usual food preparation practices, for example cooking pulses or potatoes (see Table 1, page 287).

One group of compounds worth discussing is phytates.[13] Phytates are found in almost all plants, but are particularly plentiful in whole grains, pulses, nuts and seeds. Given that whole grains and pulses only became a prominent feature in foodways after the agricultural revolution, phytates were not an issue in ancestral foodways based on fresh, wild plants and animals.[(212)]

Phytates serve an important purpose of preventing a seed (i.e. a pulse, grain, nut) from germinating until the conditions are best to support growth. Over centuries, many traditional societies have cultivated practices that reduce the amounts of phytates in food (though in the main they did so to improve flavour and/or reduce cooking time, rather than to make them more nutritious). The more that plant foods are relied on for nourishment, the more attention should be paid to using these traditional food preparation practices.

---

13   Phytate is a name for a group of compounds, including phytic acid and its related salts. Phytates are the main way that mature seeds store phosphorus. In contrast, vegetables, fruits, starchy roots and tubers are low in phytate, and animal foods contain none.

TABLE 1. COMMON ANTI-NUTRIENTS AND PRACTICES TO REDUCE THEM [213]

Anti-nutrient	Foods	Possible effect	Reduced by
Oxalates	Spinach, silverbeet (Swiss chard), sorrel, beetroot and beet greens, rhubarb, nuts, pulses, whole grains, potatoes, sweet potatoes	Reduce calcium absorption	Soaking Boiling Steaming
Phytates	Pulses, whole grains, nuts, seeds	Reduce iron, zinc, calcium and magnesium absorption	Soaking Souring (fermenting) Sprouting (germinating) Boiling
Tannins	Tea, coffee, grapes, berries, apples, stone fruit, nuts, beans, whole grains	Reduce iron absorption	Cooking Peeling skins off fruit and nuts
Goitrogens	Brassica vegetables, millet	Reduce iodine absorption	Steaming Boiling

Unpicking

The conservationist John Muir once said, 'When we try to pick out anything by itself, we find it hitched to everything else in the universe.' That is exactly how we might feel after this little exploration of the social life of nutrients. But for me, nutrition only makes sense viewed through a lens of evolutionary ecology — an appreciation for where we have come from and how that has shaped us to be who we are today. If nutrition science is to be helpful in fostering foodways that are to be healthy and sustainable, then it is to be less about individual nutrients and more about the relations between us and our deepest pasts, and in the connection between our foodways and our bodies today.

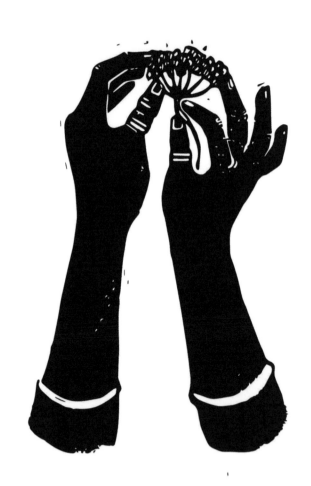

Chapter 9

ASSIST

For millions of years, humans have walked the Earth without the assistance of nutritional supplements to meet their bodies' needs. It should be perfectly possible to thrive on the three foundations of food, water and sunshine alone. However, modern lifeways mean there are some instances when nutritional supplements may assist with more quickly and easily restoring depletions or meeting raised biological needs.

Understanding Supplements

Nutritional needs ebb and flow throughout life. Sometimes our bodies need more nourishment, sometimes less. Pregnancy and breastfeeding are notable seasons of motherhood that place high demands on a woman, and nutritional depletions can also interfere with fertility. If you are having difficulty conceiving, with no obvious cause found through investigation with your doctor, then paying attention to nourishing yourself and your partner, including thinking about whether supplements may offer support, is worthwhile.

Our bodies can also be remarkably resilient and adaptable to changing needs — they have had to be. Across history, there will have been times when our ancestors made do with less food and at other times, abundance, and these experiences are woven into our bodies. All that said, making do may not be without health consequences for a mother or baby. Whatever the reason, when it is hard to meet nutritional needs through food alone, supplements may offer the possibility of plugging gaps in the short term.

Beyond the physical demands of growing a baby, instances when food intakes may fall short of nutritional needs could include severe morning sickness or prolonged illness. Or sometimes we seem to eat well, but the soils from which our food is grown may have been depleted of nutrients for various reasons, including industrial agricultural practices. Or animals may eat diets that are distant from their ancestors — changing the composition of the meat, milk and eggs as a consequence. Fruits and vegetables may be

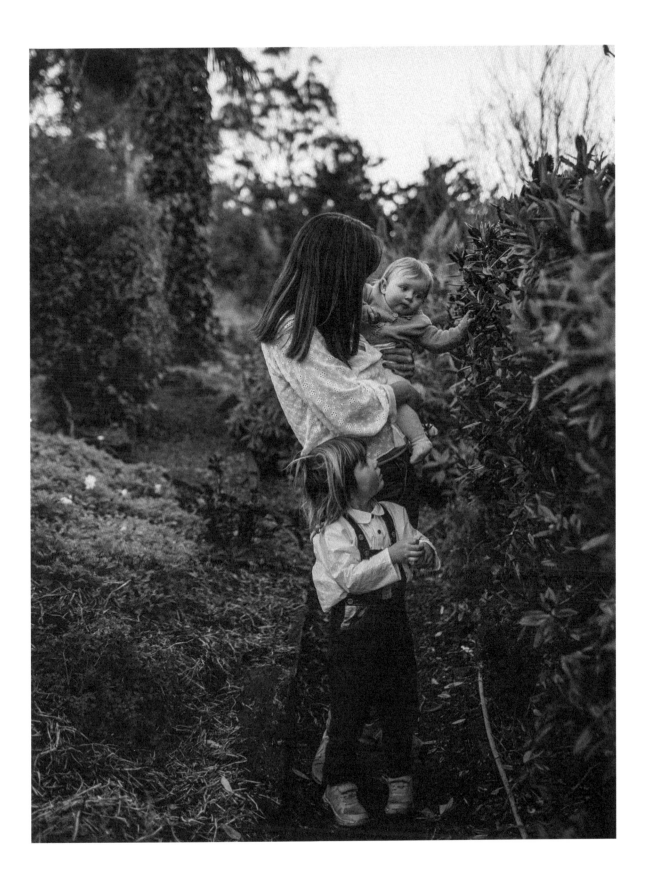

stored for long periods, gradually depleting their sensitive nutrients. And, sometimes, food intakes don't fall short, but underlying health issues may reduce the absorption of nutrients from food.

The challenge lies not in appreciating that there can be shortfalls in nutrient intakes, but in knowing whether gaps are a possibility (often without invasive medical tests), why these emerge, and whether they matter in the grand scheme of things. We should also be mindful of the limitations of isolated nutrient supplements in fulfilling roles of nourishing foods, in all their wonderful complexity.

The global nutritional supplement industry is worth over AU$200 billion annually. It has a vested interest in convincing us, through marketing and the funding of biased research, that their products offer solutions to issues that often don't even exist. In reality, supplements are not superior to foods and the likelihood of supplements being helpful is only a possibility when food intakes are inadequate (whatever the reason for that may be). When women are well nourished, there is no evidence to suggest that supplements will increase the chance of conceiving, carrying to term, or improving the health of a mother or a baby.

We begin here by looking at supplements that may be worth considering, in general, throughout the period of pre-conception, pregnancy, breastfeeding, plus before and beyond these times. The first of these is vitamin D, which may be important, depending on where people live and the amount of UVB sunlight they get. Then there are several nutrients to be mindful of when eating fewer animal foods such as B12, iodine, and some others. Following on, we explore the early stages of motherhood and look at which supplements could provide important extra assistance or insurance. These include folate in the pre-conceptual period and first trimester, and iron in middle to late pregnancy and postpartum.

Vitamin D

Vitamin D is essential throughout the pre- and peripartum periods. Before conception, vitamin D is involved in the assembly and rhythmic release of sex hormones. It also supports fertilisation and successful implantation.[214] The likelihood of conceiving with assisted conception treatment is much higher in women with adequate vitamin D levels, compared with women who are deficient.[215, 216] In men, vitamin D affects sperm quality, quantity and motility, and protects sperm DNA from damage. During pregnancy, vitamin D plays a role in relaxing the immune system so that a woman's body does not reject paternal DNA.

If you have adequate vitamin D levels, there is no evidence that supplements have any beneficial effect on fertility or pregnancy outcomes.[217] However, vitamin D deficiency is very common — on average it is evident in two-thirds of pregnancies; more in darker-skinned women.[218] This is because while it is possible to get some vitamin D from foods, particularly fish, it is very hard to fully meet needs this way. This is especially the case during pregnancy and breastfeeding when higher amounts are needed to support a baby's rapid bone growth.

We rely primarily on sunshine for vitamin D. Depending on the amount of sunshine you are exposed to (also allowing for sunscreen and clothing), as well as your skin colour, a supplement may be needed to ensure you get adequate amounts. Left untreated, vitamin D deficiency can reduce fertility and contribute to a host of long-term health issues for a mother and baby.

If you are known to be of at risk of vitamin D deficiency, supplement with vitamin D as follows: 10 µg/day in winter months, and year-round in vulnerable groups, including during pregnancy and breastfeeding.[219, 220]

Supplements for Plant-based Eating

Most of the evolutionary changes that shaped human physiology, and therefore our nutritional needs, occurred during the 2.5 million-year-long Pleistocene epoch. For almost, if not the entirety of this period, our ancestors were omnivorous — meaning that humans are biologically suited to eating a combination of plant and animal foods. Animals concentrate

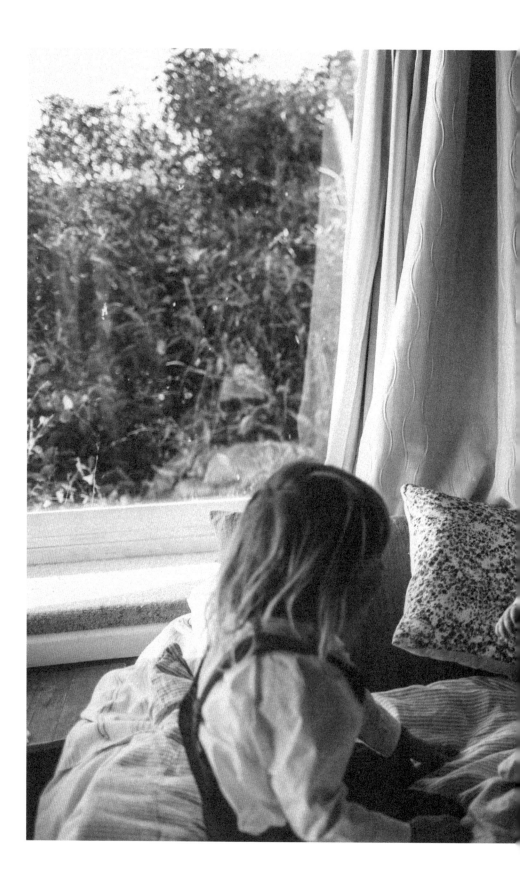

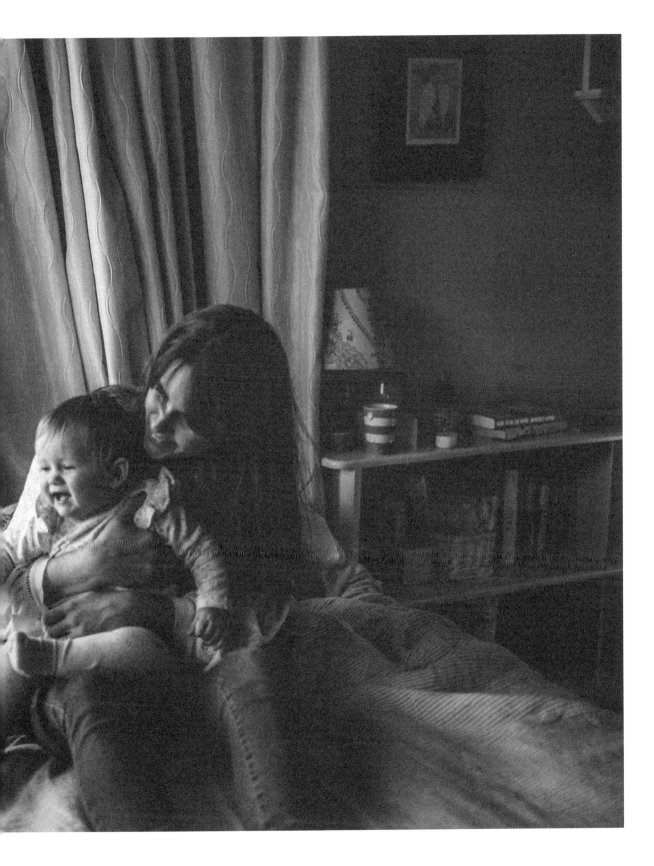

nutrients in their organs and tissues, so eating some animal foods can make it easier to meet nutritional needs, especially at times when requirements are higher.

There are a handful of nutrients that may be absent in plant foods (e.g. B12, retinol, long chain omega-3 fats), present in lower amounts than animal foods (e.g. essential amino acids), less readily absorbed (e.g. some minerals) or less widely available (e.g. iodine). However, eating few or no animal foods does not necessarily mean supplements are needed to cover all nutritional bases, nor does it mean that plant-based foodways are inferior. On the contrary, there are many studies to show that populations who eat mostly wholesome plant foods live longer, healthier lives.

Vitamin B12

Humans have evolved to need only very small amounts of B12 — the body is very efficient at recycling it and can store good amounts in the liver. Only animal foods contain B12, and the meat and organs of land animals, fish and seafood contain considerably more B12 than foods made from milk, like cheese or yoghurt, or eggs. Eating small amounts of animal foods regularly should provide enough B12. Needs only increase very slightly with pregnancy and breastfeeding, such that slightly bigger portions in line with increased appetite are a good idea at this time. However, if no animal foods are eaten, or are eaten in lesser amounts or less frequently than this, then a B12 supplement or B12 fortified products will be required (see also Micronutrients — Vitamin B12, page 272).

Iodine

Aside from sea vegetables, the iodine content of plants is generally low. If little in the way of fish, seafood or sea vegetables, milk or milk products (which are adventitiously high in iodine), or iodised salt is eaten, then iodine needs will not be met. This is especially the case during pregnancy and breastfeeding, when iodine needs are higher. In Australia, even though salt is iodised, it is recommended that across the pre- and peripartum period, women take an iodine supplement of 150 μg a day.[221] Kelp or seaweed supplements should be avoided as they can contain excessive amounts of iodine.

Omega-3

The long chain fat DHA is the most abundant omega-3 fat in the brain, eyes and nervous system. It is particularly important during pregnancy and the first couple of years of infancy, as this is when most brain development happens. There are no plant foods that contain the long chain omega-3 fats DHA and EPA. Eggs and grass-fed meat contain small amounts, but levels are considerably lower than found in oily fish. Foodways that do not include fish or do so only occasionally (less than once a week) will contain little to no long chain omega-3 fats.

Plant-based foodways contain much lower amounts of long chain omega-3 fats, or none at all in the case of vegans. This can lower the amount of these same fats in breast milk. However, while the breast milk of vegan or vegetarian mothers may contain fewer long chain omega-3 fats, it is not entirely devoid of them. A mother can draw upon her own reserve that she has assembled from shorter chain omega-3 fats.[222, 223] Whether lower intakes of long chain omega-3s matters is debated in the scientific community, because there is not good evidence in this space. Until we have more clarity, if fish is eaten less than once a week, a long chain omega-3 supplement (DHA) is a prudent choice. Algal oils are available, and these may be a more sustainable choice than supplements derived from fish.

Vitamin A

Plants do not contain retinol, the bioactive form of vitamin A. However, brightly coloured vegetables, for example carrots, squash, sweet potatoes, dark leafy greens, and to a lesser extent, colourful fruits — apricots, mango, rockmelon — contain appreciable amounts of compounds called carotenes, that the body can convert to retinol. Providing colourful produce is eaten at most meals and larger portions of these foods are eaten when pregnant and if breastfeeding, vitamin A levels should not be an issue, even with exclusively plant-based foodways. If supplements are needed, it is important to note that unlike carotenes, vitamin A in its retinol form can be teratogenic. Pregnancy supplements are specially formulated to exclude vitamin A or use beta-carotene in its place. Cod liver oil is high in retinol and should be avoided in pregnancy.

Minerals

Minerals such as calcium, iron and zinc are often present in plant foods. In fact, studies of vegetarian and vegan populations generally show that they have higher intakes of these minerals.[224] However, while intakes may be higher with plant-based eating, the amounts that are absorbed can vary considerably depending on whole diet and food practices. In other words, higher mineral intakes do not necessarily mean that needs are met. The inclusion of mineral promoters (e.g. vitamin C in fruit) and mineral inhibitors (e.g. tannins in tea and coffee) will affect things (see also Anti-nutrients, page 285). Foodways that are based on whole plant foods, abundant in fresh fruit and vegetables, and that make use of traditional food preparation practices, should provide enough in the way of minerals.

Pre-conception

Folate

Given the essential role of folate in DNA assembly, it is crucial during pregnancy; especially in the early stages, when cells are rapidly proliferating, and body parts are forming. Insufficient folate can affect development and cause birth defects including spina bifida, which arises when the neural tube does not close properly in the first four weeks of pregnancy.[225] However, even before conception, impaired folate status can affect fertility by disrupting ovulation and reducing egg quality. Improving folate intakes, if they are low, can enhance fertility and increase the likelihood of and reduce the overall time to pregnancy.[226]

Folate must be obtained from food. It is perfectly possible to get adequate amounts when routinely eating fresh, colourful vegetables, especially dark leafy greens, and pulses and whole grains. However, folate is a relatively unstable nutrient, meaning levels can reduce considerably with exposure to light and high temperatures (above 100°C). It also leaches easily into cooking water and is lost that way, unless the water is consumed as well (as with soup).

For these reasons, folate supplementation is recommended for at least four weeks before pregnancy and throughout the first trimester. However, because it can take several weeks to replete folate stores and many women become pregnant without active planning, over eighty countries worldwide have laws that require staple manufactured foods, such as bread, to be fortified with folic acid, the synthetic version of folate.[227] Some other countries, including the UK and Ireland, have hesitated to follow suit, largely over concerns around exposure to high levels of unmetabolised folic acid in the blood.

When choosing a supplement, it is preferable to choose the bioactive form 5-methyltetrahydrofolate (5-MTHF), rather than folic acid, as the latter needs to undergo several metabolic steps to make it usable.[228–230] Some people can carry a gene variant (usually unknowingly) which affects their ability to convert folic acid to folate.[231] Incidentally, one of these variants (known as the C677T) is the most well-established genetic risk factor for developing neural tube defects.[232]

If you are planning to conceive or are pregnant, supplement with folate as follows: 400 mg/d at least four weeks before conception and continue until 12 weeks pregnant.

Note that women at risk of B12 deficiency who are hoping to conceive or who are pregnant already should not have folate supplementation alone without B12.[233] This is because folate can do some of the same jobs as B12, apart from nerve protection. In cases of B12 deficiency, folate can hide nerve damage.

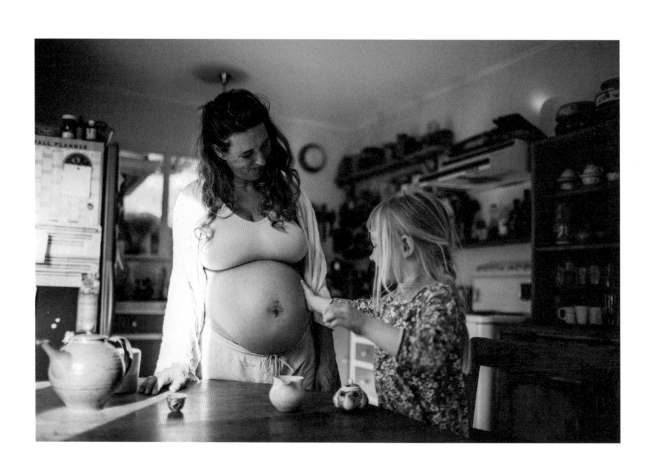

Pregnancy

Vitamin B6

Some studies have found that supplementing with vitamin B6 can help alleviate morning sickness, although it is unclear why this would be the case.[234] Pregnancy markedly reduces B6 levels in a woman as the nutrient is transferred to the baby. However, it is unclear whether B6 needs during pregnancy should increase to offset this. Even so, intakes of B6 are generally not a concern as it is abundant in whole plant foods, including green leafy vegetables, whole grains and pulses. It is also found in meat, fish, eggs and dairy foods. Bacteria in the lower gut can also make B6, which is also where it can be absorbed from.

Folate

Routine folate supplementation should be continued until the end of the first trimester. If folate supplements have not been taken before pregnancy, folate stores can be raised quickly, prior to neural tube closure at 28 days after conception, using the following regimen:

7500 mg (7.5 mg) 5-MTHF once a day for four days (four doses) or 7500 mg (7.5 mg) 5-MTHF twice a day (every 12 hours) for two and a half days (five doses).[235]

Note that this regimen is for rapid, short-term repletion of stores only and there is no advantage to continuing at this level for the duration of your pregnancy.

Iodine

During pregnancy, more iodine is needed to support increased production of thyroid hormones.[236] However, it is unclear whether the body needs more iodine from foods (or a supplement) because it can adapt to absorb more if needed.[237, 238] The body stores iodine in the thyroid gland and controls losses well — it loses less iodine when needs are increased and more when they are not. These adaptations work to ensure a baby doesn't miss out on this essential nutrient during pregnancy.[239]

On the other hand, there are concerns that even mild iodine deficiency during pregnancy can affect a baby's cognitive development well into childhood, if not beyond.[240] As with other nutrients, there are no known benefits of supplementing with iodine during pregnancy when intakes are adequate, and even when they are not, the evidence is unclear.[241] This could perhaps be due to the fact that building nutritional status takes time. If you are at risk of low iodine levels, it is worth considering a supplement (see also Supplements for Plant-based Eating, page 293).

Iron

Although less iron is needed early on in pregnancy than beforehand (because menstruation stops), after the first trimester, iron requirements increase significantly.[242] Iron is critical to sustaining a baby's rapid growth, particularly of their brain. So much so that a woman's body prioritises transferring iron to her baby, at the expense of meeting her own needs.[243] While this can mean that pregnancy can increase the risk of iron deficiency and anaemia, unless these are diagnosed,[14] supplementation is unnecessary and potentially harmful in women with adequate or near-adequate iron levels.[244]

Supplemental iron in pregnancy can be problematic in several ways. Firstly, despite iron being essential for life, free iron is toxic to the body and concerns have been raised that in excess it can be teratogenic in the first trimester.[245] Excess iron in the digestive tract can also create gut disturbances like constipation, nausea and vomiting. In the first instance, the focus should primarily be on eating more iron-rich foods and using practices that promote absorption, rather than having a supplement.

---

14   A blood test is needed to confirm if low iron levels are present.

Postpartum

Pregnancy and birth may leave a woman nutritionally depleted, especially if excessive blood loss is experienced (some women may receive a blood transfusion, but others do not). Breastfeeding can also be the most nutritionally demanding phase in a woman's life, even more so than pregnancy. During the first four to six months of life, a baby will double the weight gained during the entire nine months of pregnancy. Eating well at this time ensures a mother's nutritional stores are not depleted at the expense of producing breast milk, which is incredibly rich in nutrients. The duration and intensity of breastfeeding will influence the amount of food a woman needs to eat. In time, nourishing foodways will work to restore health but, particularly when coupled with the physically draining early days and weeks of postpartum, some may be interested in supplements that could quicken nutritional repletion.

Iron

Pregnancy, blood loss during birth, and postpartum lochia may all drain a woman's iron reserves, and this can exacerbate the feelings of tiredness and lethargy that are common in the newborn phase. Nevertheless, this may not mean that iron supplements are needed. In contrast to pregnancy, postpartum iron needs are relatively low, even when breastfeeding. This is partly due to the continued cessation of menses (lactational amenorrhoea), which can extend for six months with exclusive breastfeeding, if not longer.

Newborns also need significantly less iron than during pregnancy. Iron in breast milk is combined with a special protein called *lactoferrin* which ensures it is readily absorbed. While the iron level in breast milk is much lower than formula, babies absorb about 50 per cent of it, compared to only 10 per cent absorbed from formula.[246] The amount of iron in breast milk is tightly regulated and does not vary according to a mother's iron status.[247] If you are concerned about your iron levels you can request a blood test from your doctor and commence supplementation if indicated.

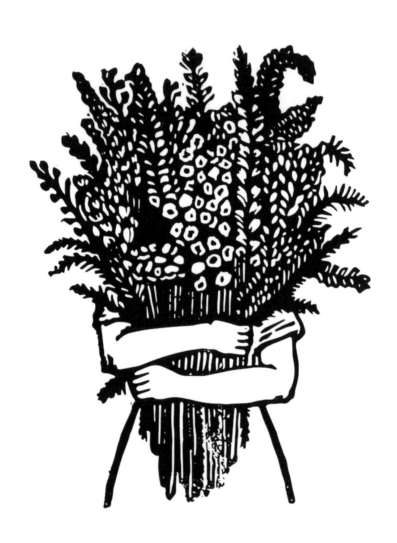

Conclusion

COMING
TOGETHER

Food offers uncountable connections to our world. As we pay closer attention to our way of food and how our practices relate to ourselves, each other and the Earth, we will begin the important work of healing the rift between humans and the Earth. For there is little else I can think of that so intimately binds us to one another, as growing food, preparing and sharing it with others, and taking it into our bodies. Food is the rare thread that is woven through the fabric of life.

Awakened to our reality, our task now, knowing what we do, is to nourish each other, in spite of the systems around us that would have us do otherwise. From my own experience, I believe that with the transition to motherhood comes an invitation to rematriate our foodways and to realise our strength and creative capacity to shape nourishing foodways that will nurture us and the generations that follow.

Motherhood also quietly teaches us to let go of our preconceptions of how things will be and know that life is full of possibilities. Walking on, we cannot know what lies ahead. We can only live with our questions and learn how to slow down and listen for the whispers of answers that may come from the most surprising places. One of which will almost certainly be the unbounded minds of our children.

Our children jolt us with a force that has the power to transform our way of seeing and experiencing the world, whether we think we are ready for it, or not. As Bucky Fuller once said, 'there is nothing in a caterpillar that tells you it's going to be a butterfly' — and so welcome, dear caterpillar, onto this uncharted path of unravelling and reweaving — who knows where it may lead.

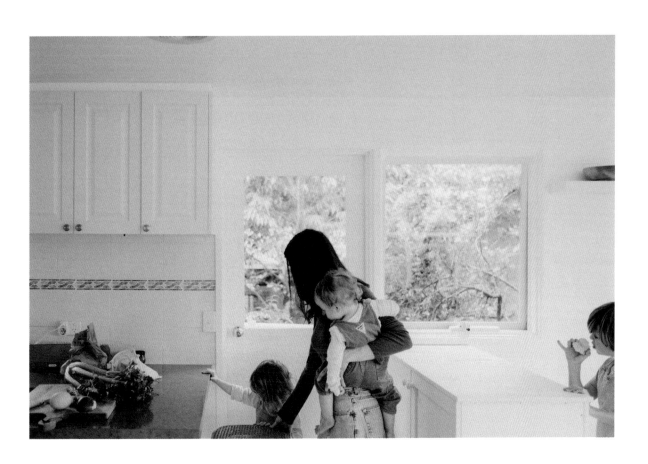

ENDNOTES

1. Kuipers RS, Luxwolda MF, Janneke Dijck-Brouwer DA, Eaton SB, Crawford MA, Cordain L, et al. Estimated Macronutrient and Fatty Acid Intakes from an East African Paleolithic Diet. *British Journal of Nutrition*. 2010;104(11):1666–87.
2. Richerson PJ, Boyd R, Bettinger RL. Was Agriculture Impossible During the Pleistocene but Mandatory During the Holocene? A Climate Change Hypothesis. *American Antiquity*. 2001;66(3):387–411.
3. Pascoe B. *Dark Emu: Aboriginal Australia and the Birth of Agriculture*. Magabala Books; 2018.
4. Winson A, Choi JY. Dietary Regimes and the Nutrition Transition: Bridging Disciplinary Domains. *Agriculture and Human Values*. 2017;34(3):559–72.
5. Book UY. *Emerging Issues in our Global Environment*. United Nations Environment Programme, Nairobi. 2011.
6. Hemler EC, Hu FB. Plant-Based Diets for Personal, Population, and Planetary Health. *Advances in Nutrition*. 2019;10(Supplement_4):S275–S83.
7. Poore J, Nemecek T. Reducing Food's Environmental Impacts Through Producers and Consumers. *Science*. 2018;360(6392):987–92.
8. DL. K. Paleo for a Shrinking Planet? Huffington Post [Internet]; 19 February, 2015 [Available from: https://www.huffpost.com/entry/paleo-for-a-shrinking-pla_b_6712936.]
9. Bronson FH. Are Humans Seasonally Photoperiodic? *Journal of Biological Rhythms*. 2004;19(3):180–92.
10. Muscogiuri G, Altieri B, de Angelis C, Palomba S, Pivonello R, Colao A, et al. Shedding New Light on Female Fertility: The Role of Vitamin D. *Reviews in Endocrine and Metabolic Disorders*. 2017;18(3):273–83.
11. FAO. *The Second Report on the State of the World's Plant Genetic Resources for Food and Agriculture*. Rome: Food and Agriculture Organisation; 2010.
12. Ibid.
13. Khoury CK, Bjorkman AD, Dempewolf H, Ramirez-Villegas J, Guarino L, Jarvis A, et al. Increasing Homogeneity in Global Food Supplies and the Implications for Food Security. *Proceedings of the National Academy of Sciences*. 2014;111(11):4001.
14. Zimmerer KS, de Haan S, Jones AD, Creed-Kanashiro H, Tello M, Carrasco M, et al. The Biodiversity of Food and Agriculture (Agrobiodiversity) in the Anthropocene: Research Advances and Conceptual Framework. *Anthropocene*. 2019;25:100192.
15. Simonyte Sjödin K, Vidman L, Rydén P, West CE. Emerging Evidence of the Role of Gut Microbiota in the Development of Allergic Diseases. *Current Opinion in Allergy and Clinical Immunology*. 2016;16(4):390–5.
16. Ibid.
17. Friedmann H. Towards a Natural History of Foodgetting. *Sociologia Ruralis*. 2017;57(2):245– 64.
18. Wagner DL. Insect Declines in the Anthropocene. *Annual Review of Entomology*. 2020;65(1):457–80.
19. Chiu YH, Afeiche MC, Gaskins AJ, Williams PL, Petrozza JC, Tanrikut C, et al. Fruit and Vegetable Intake and their Pesticide Residues in Relation to Semen Quality Among Men from a Fertility Clinic. *Human Reproduction*. 2015;30(6):1342–51.

20. Gore AC, Chappell VA, Fenton SE, Flaws JA, Nadal A, Prins GS, et al. EDC-2: The Endocrine Society's Second Scientific Statement on Endocrine-Disrupting Chemicals. *Endocrine Reviews*. 2015;36(6):E1–E150.
21. Robinson J. *Eating on the Wild Side*. New York: Little, Brown and Company; 2013.
22. Ludwig DS, Hu FB, Tappy L, Brand-Miller J. Dietary Carbohydrates: Role of Quality and Quantity in Chronic Disease. *BMJ*. 2018;361:k2340.
23. Gibson RS, Raboy V, King JC. Implications of Phytate in Plant-based Foods for Iron and Zinc Bioavailability, Setting Dietary Requirements, and Formulating Programs and Policies. *Nut Rev*. 2018;76(11):793–804.
24. Gibson RS, Donovan UM, Heath AL. Dietary Strategies to Improve the Iron and Zinc Nutriture of Young Women Following a Vegetarian Diet. *Plant Foods Hum Nutr*. 1997;51(1):1–16.
25. Schlemmer U, Frølich W, Prieto RM, Grases F. Phytate in Foods and Significance for Humans: Food Sources, Intake, Processing, Bioavailability, Protective Role and Analysis. *Mol Nutr Food Res*. 2009;53(2):S330–75.
26. Katz S. *The Art of Fermentation*. Vermont: Chelsea Green Publishing; 2012.
27. Mariotti Lippi M, Foggi B, Aranguren B, Ronchitelli A, Revedin A. Multistep Food Plant Processing at Grotta Paglicci (Southern Italy) around 32,600 cal B.P. *Proceedings of the National Academy of Sciences*. 2015;112(39):12075.
28. Mercader J. Mozambican Grass Seed Consumption During the Middle Stone Age. *Science*. 2009;326(5960):1680.
29. Salazar C, García-Cárdenas JM, Paz-y-Miño C. Understanding Celiac Disease from Genetics to the Future Diagnostic Strategies. *Clinical Medicine Insights: Gastroenterology*. 2017;10:1179552217712249.
30. Cheng M-H, Sekhon JJK, Rosentrater KA, Wang T, Jung S, Johnson LA. Environmental Impact Assessment of Soybean Oil Production: Extruding-expelling Process, Hexane Extraction and Aqueous Extraction. *Food and Bioproducts Processing*. 2018;108:58–68.
31. Kumar SPJ, Prasad SR, Banerjee R, Agarwal DK, Kulkarni KS, Ramesh KV. Green Solvents and Technologies for Oil Extraction from Oilseeds. *Chem Cent J*. 2017;11:9.
32. Ong H-T, Samsudin H, Soto-Valdez H. Migration of Endocrine-disrupting Chemicals into Food from Plastic Packaging Materials: An Overview of Chemical Risk Assessment, Techniques to Monitor Migration, and International Regulations. *Critical Reviews in Food Science and Nutrition*. 2020;1–23.
33. Neelakantan N, Seah Jowy Yi H, van Dam Rob M. The Effect of Coconut Oil Consumption on Cardiovascular Risk Factors. *Circulation*. 2020;141(10):803–14.
34. Eyres L, Eyres MF, Chisholm A, Brown RC. Coconut Oil Consumption and Cardiovascular Risk Factors in Humans. *Nutr Rev*. 2016;74(4):267–80.
35. Galili E, Langgut D, Terral JF, Barazani O, Dag A, Kolska Horwitz L, et al. Early Production of Table Olives at a Mid-7th Millennium BP Submerged Site Off the Carmel Coast (Israel). *Sci Rep*. 2021;11(1):2218.
36. Cazzolla Gatti R, Liang J, Velichevskaya A, Zhou M. Sustainable Palm Oil May Aot be so Sustainable. *Science of The Total Environment*. 2019;652:48–51.
37. Pye O. Commodifying Sustainability: Development, Nature and Politics in the Palm Oil Industry. *World Development*. 2019;121:218–28.
38. Ludwig DS, Ebbeling CB. The Carbohydrate-Insulin Model of Obesity: Beyond 'Calories In, Calories Out'. *JAMA Intern Med*. 2018;178(8):1098–103.
39. Barclay A, Sandall, P, Shwide-Slavin, C. *The Ultimate Guide to Sugars and Sweeteners*. New York: The Experiment; 2014.
40. Russell C, Grimes C, Baker P, Sievert K, Lawrence MA. The Drivers, Trends and Dietary Impacts of Non-nutritive Sweeteners in the Food Supply: A Narrative Review. *Nutrition Research Reviews*. 2020;1–67.
41. Ruiz-Ojeda FJ, Plaza-Díaz J, Sáez-Lara MJ, Gil A. Effects of Sweeteners on the Gut Microbiota: A Review of Experimental Studies and Clinical Trials. *Adv Nutr*. 2019;10(suppl_1):S31–S48.
42. Li D, O'Brien JW, Tscharke BJ, Choi PM, Zheng Q, Ahmed F, et al. National Wastewater Reconnaissance of Artificial Sweetener Consumption and Emission in Australia. *Environment International*. 2020;143:105963.
43. Lyngsø J, Ramlau-Hansen CH, Bay B, Ingerslev HJ, Hulman A, Kesmodel US. Association Between Coffee or Caffeine Consumption and Fecundity and Fertility: A Systematic Review and Dose-response Meta-analysis. *Clin Epidemiol*. 2017;9:699–719.
44. Ricci E, Viganò P, Cipriani S, Somigliana E, Chiaffarino F, Bulfoni A, et al. Coffee and Caffeine Intake and Male Infertility: A Systematic Review. *Nutr J*. 2017;16(1):37.
45. Lyngsø. Association Between Coffee or Caffeine Consumption and Fecundity and Fertility. *Clin Epidemiol*. 699–719.

46. EFSA Panel on Dietetic Products. Scientific Opinion on the Safety of Caffeine. *EFSA J.* 2015;13(5):4102.

47. McCreedy A, Bird S, Brown LJ, Shaw-Stewart J, Chen YF. Effects of Maternal Caffeine Consumption on the Breastfed Child: A Systematic Review. *Swiss Med Wkly.* 2018;28(148):w14665.

48. de Angelis CA-OX, Nardone A, Garifalos F, Pivonello C, Sansone A, Conforti A, et al. Smoke, Alcohol and Drug Addiction and Female Fertility. *Rep Bio Endo.* 2020;18(21).

49. Van Heertum KA-O, Rossi B. Alcohol and Fertility: How Much is Too Much? *Fertil Res Pract.* 2017;3(10).

50. Jenkins DJA, Sievenpiper JL, Pauly D, Sumaila UR, Kendall CWC, Mowat FM. Are Dietary Recommendations for the Use of Fish Oils Sustainable? *Canadian Medical Association Journal.* 2009;180(6):633.

51. Naylor RL, Goldburg RJ, Primavera JH, Kautsky N, Beveridge MCM, Clay J, et al. Effect of Aquaculture on World Fish Supplies. *Nature.* 2000;405(6790):1017–24.

52. Jenkins. Are Dietary Recommendations for the Use of Fish Oils Sustainable? *Canadian Medical Association Journal.* 633.

53. Hemler. Plant-Based Diets for Personal, Population, and Planetary Health. *Advances in Nutrition.* S275–S83.

54. Smil V. Eating Meat: Evolution, Patterns, and Consequences. Population and Development Review. 2002;28(4):599–639.

55. Machovina B, Feeley KJ, Ripple WJ. Biodiversity Conservation: The Key is Reducing Meat Consumption. *Science of The Total Environment.* 2015;536:419–31.

56. Ibid.

57. Thornton A. This is How Many Animals We Eat Each Year 2019 [Available from: https://www.weforum.org/agenda/2019/02/chart-of-the-day-this-is-how-many-animals-we-eat-each- year/.]

58. D'Silva J. Adverse Impact of Industrial Animal Agriculture on the Health and Welfare of Farmed Animals. *Integrative Zoology.* 2006;1(1):53–8.

59. Ibid.

60. Vallianou NA-O, Dalamaga M, Stratigou T, Karampela I, Tsigalou C. Do Antibiotics Cause Obesity Through Long-term Alterations in the Gut Microbiome? *A Review of Current Evidence. Curr Obes Rep.* 2021;10(3):244–62.

61. Willett W, Rockström J, Loken B, Springmann M, Lang T, Vermeulen S, et al. Food in the Anthropocene: the EAT–Lancet Commission on Healthy Diets from Sustainable Food Systems. *The Lancet.* 2019;393(10170):447–92.

62. Stoll-Kleemann S, O'Riordan T. The Sustainability Challenges of Our Meat and Dairy Diets. *Environment: Science and Policy for Sustainable Development.* 2015;57(3):34–48.

63. Hemler. Plant-Based Diets for Personal, Population, and Planetary Health. *Advances in Nutrition.* S275–S83.

64. Altieri MA, Nicholls CI. Agroecology Scaling Up for Food Sovereignty and Resiliency. In: Lichtfouse E, editor. Sustainable Agriculture Reviews: Volume 11. Dordrecht: Springer Netherlands; 2012. p. 1–29.

65. Wells JCK. Commentary: Paternal and Maternal Influences on Offspring Phenotype: the Same, Only Different. *International Journal of Epidemiology.* 2014;43(3):772–4.

66. Lane M, Robker RL, Robertson SA. Parenting from Before Conception. *Science.* 2014;345(6198):756.

67. Fleming TP, Watkins AJ, Velazquez MA, Mathers JC, Prentice AM, Stephenson J, et al. Origins of Lifetime Health Around the Time of Conception: Causes and Consequences. *The Lancet.* 2018;391(10132):1842–52.

68. Stephenson J, Heslehurst N, Hall J, Schoenaker DAJM, Hutchinson J, Cade JE, et al. Before the Beginning: Nutrition and Lifestyle in the Preconception Period and its Importance for Future Health. *The Lancet.* 2018;391(10132):1830–41.

69. Choy JT, Eisenberg ML. Male Infertility as a Window to Health. *Fertility and Sterility.* 2018;110(5):810–4.

70. Chavarro JE, Rich-Edwards JW, Rosner BA, Willett WC. Diet and Lifestyle in the Prevention of Ovulatory Disorder Infertility. *Obstetrics & Gynecology.* 2007;110(5).

71. Firns S, Cruzat VF, Keane KN, Joesbury KA, Lee AH, Newsholme P, et al. The Effect of Cigarette Smoking, Alcohol Consumption and Fruit and Vegetable Consumption on IVF Outcomes: A Review and Presentation of Original Data. *Reprod Biol Endocrinol.* 2015;16(13):134.

72. Stephenson. Before the Beginning. *The Lancet.* 1830–41.

73. Wakeman M. A Review of the Effects of Oral Contraceptives on Nutrient Status, with Especial Consideration to Folate in UK. *Journal of Advances in Medicine and Medical Research.* 2019;1–17.

74. Miller EM. The Reproductive Ecology of Iron in Women. *Am J Phys Anthropol.* 2016;159(61):S172–96.

75. Wendt A, Gibbs CM, Peters S, Hogue CJ. Impact of Increasing Inter-pregnancy Interval on Maternal and Infant Health. *Paediatric and Perinatal Epidemiology*. 2012;26(s1):239–58.

76. Miller. The Reproductive Ecology of Iron in Women. *Am J Phys Anthropol*. S172–96.

77. Dewey KG, Cohen RJ. Does Birth Spacing Affect Maternal or Child Nutritional Status? A Systematic Literature Review. *Matern Child Nutr*. 2007;3(3):151–73.

78. Critchley HOD, Babayev E, Bulun SE, Clark S, Garcia-Grau I, Gregersen PK, et al. Menstruation: Science and Society. *American Journal of Obstetrics & Gynecology*. 2020;223(5):624–64.

79. Lyngsø. Association Between Coffee or Caffeine Consumption and Fecundity and Fertility. *Clin Epidemiol*. 699–719.

80. Moghetti PA-O, Tosi F. Insulin Resistance and PCOS: Chicken or Egg? *J Endocrinol Invest*. 2021;44(2):233–44.

81. Muscogiuri. Shedding New Light on Female Fertility. *Reviews in Endocrine and Metabolic Disorders*. 273–83.

82. Lerchbaum E, Rabe T. Vitamin D and Female Fertility. *Current Opinion in Obstetrics and Gynecology*. 2014;26(3).

83. Barrea L, Marzullo P, Muscogiuri G, Di Somma C, Scacchi M, Orio F, et al. Source and Amount of Carbohydrate in the Diet and Inflammation in Women with Polycystic Ovary Syndrome. *Nutrition Research Reviews*. 2018;31(2):291–301.

84. Hart MJ, Torres SJ, McNaughton SA, Milte CM. Dietary Patterns and Associations with Biomarkers of Inflammation in Adults: A Systematic Review of Observational Studies. *Nutr J*. 2021;20(1):24.

85. Willis SK, Wise LA, Wesselink AK, Rothman KJ, Mikkelsen EM, Tucker KL, et al. Glycemic Load, Dietary Fiber, and Added Sugar and Fecundability in 2 Preconception Cohorts. *Am J Clin Nutr*. 2020;112(1):27–38.

86. Critchley. Menstruation. *American Journal of Obstetrics & Gynecology*. 624–64.

87. Garcia-Fernandez J, García-Velasco JA. Endometriosis and Reproduction: What We Have Learned. *Yale J Biol Med*. 2020;93(4):571–77.

88. Huijs E, Nap A. The Effects of Nutrients on Symptoms in Women with Endometriosis: A Systematic Review. *Reproductive BioMedicine Online*. 2020;41(2):317–28.

89. Chiaffarino FA-O, Cipriani S, Ricci E, Mauri PA, Esposito G, Barretta M, et al. Endometriosis and Irritable Bowel Syndrome: A Systematic Review and Meta-analysis. *Arch Gynecol Obstet*. 2021;303(1):17–25.

90. Saguyod SJU, Kelley AS, Velarde MC, Simmen RCM. Diet and Endometriosis — Revisiting the Linkages to Inflammation. *Journal of Endometriosis and Pelvic Pain Disorders*. 2018;10(2):51–8.

91. Simmen RCM, Kelley AS. Seeing Red: Diet and Endometriosis risk. *Ann Transl Med*. 2018;6(Suppl 2):S119–S.

92. Yamamoto A, Harris HR, Vitonis AF, Chavarro JE, Missmer SA. A Prospective Cohort Study of Meat and Fish Consumption and Endometriosis Risk. *American Journal of Obstetrics & Gynecology*. 2018;219(2):178.e1–.e10.

93. Critchley. Menstruation *American Journal of Obstetrics & Gynecology*. 624–64.

94. Ibid.

95. Critchley. Menstruation. *American Journal of Obstetrics & Gynecology*. 624–64.

96. Levine H, Jørgensen N, Martino-Andrade A, Mendiola J, Weksler-Derri D, Mindlis I, et al. Temporal Trends in Sperm Count: A Systematic Review and Meta-regression Analysis. *Hum Reprod Update*. 2017;23(6):646–59.

97. Agarwal A, Mulgund A, Hamada A, Chyatte MR. A Unique View on Male Infertility Around the Globe. *Reproductive Biology and Endocrinology*. 2015;13(1):37.

98. Hayden RP, Flannigan R, Schlegel PN. The Role of Lifestyle in Male Infertility: Diet, Physical Activity, and Body Habitus. *Current Urology Reports*. 2018;19(7):56.

99. Giahi L, Mohammadmoradi S, Javidan A, Sadeghi MR. Nutritional Modifications in Male Infertility: A Systematic Review Covering 2 Decades. *Nutr Rev*. 2016;74(2):118–30.

100. Chavarro. Diet and Lifestyle in the Prevention of Ovulatory Disorder Infertility. *Obstetrics & Gynecology*.

101. Willis. Glycemic Load, Dietary Fiber, and Added Sugar and Fecundability in 2 Preconception Cohorts. *Am J Clin Nutr*. 27–38.

102. Ibid.

103. Noli SA, Ferrari S, Ricci E, Reschini M, Cipriani S, Dallagiovanna C, et al. The Role of Diet in Unexpected Poor Response to Ovarian Stimulation: A Cross-sectional Study. *Reproductive BioMedicine Online*. 2020;41(5):874–83.

104. Chavarro JE, Rich-Edwards JW, Willett WC. A Prospective Study of Dietary Carbohydrate Quantity and Quality in Relation to Risk of Ovulatory Infertility. *Eur J Clin Nutr*. 2009;63(1):78–86.

105. Chavarro JE, Rich-Edwards JW, Rosner BA, Willett WC. Protein Intake and Ovulatory Infertility. *American Journal of Obstetrics & Gynecology*. 2008;198(2):210.
106. Rolfo A, Nuzzo AM, De Amicis R, Moretti L, Bertoli S, Leone A. Fetal-Maternal Exposure to Endocrine Disruptors: Correlation with Diet Intake and Pregnancy Outcomes. *Nutrients*. 2020;12(6):1744.
107. Kahn LG, Philippat C, Nakayama SF, Slama R, Trasande L. Endocrine-disrupting Chemicals: Implications for Human Health. *Lancet Diabetes Endocrinol*. 2020;8(8):703–18.
108. Ibid.
109. Segal TR, Giudice LC. Before the Beginning: Environmental Exposures and Reproductive and Obstetrical Outcomes. *Fertility and Sterility*. 2019;112(4):613–21.
110. Mínguez-Alarcón L, Bellavia A, Gaskins AJ, Chavarro JE, Ford JB, Souter I, et al. Paternal Mixtures of Urinary Concentrations of Phthalate Metabolites, Bisphenol A and Parabens in Relation to Pregnancy Outcomes Among Couples Attending a Fertility Center. *Environ Int*. 2021;146:106171.
111. Filardi T, Panimolle F, Lenzi A, Morano S. Bisphenol A and Phthalates in Diet: An Emerging Link with Pregnancy Complications. *Nutrients*. 2020;12(2):525.
112. Geens T, Aerts D, Berthot C, Bourguignon J-P, Goeyens L, Lecomte P, Maghuin-Rogister G, et al. A Review of Dietary and Non-dietary Exposure to Bisphenol-A. *Food Chem Toxicol*. 2012:50(10).
113. Rolfo. Fetal-Maternal Exposure to Endocrine Disruptors. *Nutrients*. 1744.
114. Segal. Before the Beginning. *Fertility and Sterility*. 613–21.
115. Martínez Steele E, Khandpur N, da Costa Louzada ML, Monteiro CA. Association Between Dietary Contribution of Ultra-processed Foods and Urinary Concentrations of Phthalates and Bisphenol in a Nationally Representative Sample of the US Population Aged 6 years and Older. *PLOS ONE*. 2020;15(7):e0236738.
116. Rudel RA, Gray JM, Engel CL, Rawsthorne TW, Dodson RE, Ackerman JM, et al. Food Packaging and Bisphenol A and Bis(2-ethylhexyl) Phthalate Exposure: Findings From a Dietary Intervention. *Environ Health Perspect*. 2011;119(7):914–20.
117. Ravichandran G, Lakshmanan DK, Raju K, Elangovan A, Nambirajan G, Devanesan AA, et al. Food Advanced Glycation End Products as Potential Endocrine Disruptors: An Emerging Threat to Contemporary and Future Generations. *Environment Intl*. 2019;123:486–500.
118. Kahn. Endocrine-disrupting Chemicals. *Lancet Diabetes Endocrinol*. 703–18.
119. Brett KE, Ferraro ZM, Yockell-Lelievre J, Gruslin A, Adamo KB. Maternal-fetal Nutrient Transport in Pregnancy Pathologies: The Role of the Placenta. *Int J Mol Sci*. 2014;15(9):16153–85.
120. Young SM, Benyshek DC. In Search of Human Placentophagy: A Cross-Cultural Survey of Human Placenta Consumption, Disposal Practices, and Cultural Beliefs. *Ecology of Food and Nutrition*. 2010;49(6):467–84.
121. Koletzko B, Godfrey KM, Poston L, Szajewska H, van Goudoever JB, de Waard M, et al. Nutrition During Pregnancy, Lactation and Early Childhood and its Implications for Maternal and Long-Term Child Health: The Early Nutrition Project Recommendations. *Annals of Nutrition and Metabolism*. 2019;74(2):93–106.
122. Sherman PW, Flaxman SM. Nausea and Vomiting of Pregnancy in an Evolutionary Perspective. *Am J Obstet Gynecol*. 2002:186(5);S190–7.
123. Ibid.
124. ACOG Practice Bulletin No. 189: Nausea and Vomiting of Pregnancy. (1873–233X (Electronic)).
125. Dypvik J, Pereira AL, Tanbo TG, Eskild A. Maternal Human Chorionic Gonadotrophin Concentrations in Very Early Pregnancy and Risk of Hyperemesis Gravidarum: A Retrospective Cohort Study of 4372 Pregnancies After in Vitro Fertilization. *Eur J Obstet Gynecol Reprod Biol*. 2018;221;12–6.
126. Sherman. Nausea and Vomiting of Pregnancy in an Evolutionary Perspective. *Am J Obstet Gynecol*. S190–7.
127. Fejzo MS, Sazonova OV, Sathirapongsasuti JF, Hallgrímsdóttir IB, Vacic V, MacGibbon KW, et al. Placenta and Appetite Genes GDF15 and IGFBP7 are Associated with Hyperemesis Gravidarum. *Nature Communications*. 2018;9(1):1178.
128. Fejzo MS, Trovik J, Grooten IJ, Sridharan K, Roseboom TJ, Vikanes Å, et al. Nausea and Vomiting of Pregnancy and Hyperemesis Gravidarum. *Nature Reviews Disease Primers*. 2019;5(1):62.
129. Ibid.
130. Viljoen E, Visser J, Koen N, Musekiwa A. A Systematic Review and Meta-analysis of the Effect and Safety of Ginger in the Treatment of Pregnancy-associated Nausea and Vomiting. *Nutr J*. 2014;13:20.
131. Orloff NC, Hormes JM. Pickles and Ice Cream! Food Cravings in Pregnancy: Hypotheses, Preliminary Evidence, and Directions for Future Research. *Frontiers in Psychology*. 2014;5:1076.
132. Young SL. Pica in Pregnancy: New Ideas About an Old Condition. *Annual Review of Nutrition*. 2010;30(1):403–22.

133. Fawcett EJ, Fawcett JM, Mazmanian D. A Meta-analysis of the Worldwide Prevalence of Pica During Pregnancy and the Postpartum Period. *Int J Gyn Obstet*. 2016;133(3):277–83.

134. Zielinski R, Searing K Fau — Deibel M, Deibel M. Gastrointestinal Distress in Pregnancy: Prevalence, Assessment, and Treatment of 5 Common Minor Discomforts. *J Perinat Neonatal Nurs*. 2015;29(1):23–31.

135. Scaglione F, Panzavolta G. Folate, Folic Acid and 5-methyltetrahydrofolate are not the Same Thing. *Xenobiotica*. 2014;44(5):480–8.

136. McIntyre HD, Catalano P, Zhang C, Desoye G, Mathiesen ER, Damm P. Gestational Diabetes Mellitus. *Nature Reviews Disease Primers*. 2019;5(1):47.

137. Brett. Maternal-fetal Nutrient Transport in Pregnancy Pathologies. *Int J Mol Sci*. 16153–85.

138. McIntyre. Gestational Diabetes Mellitus. *Nature Reviews Disease Primers*. 47.

139. Fuhler GM. The Immune System and Microbiome in Pregnancy. *Best Pract Res Clin Gastroenterol*. 2020;44–5.

140. Quinete N, Schettgen T, Bertram J, Kraus T. Occurrence and Distribution of PCB Metabolites in Blood and Their Potential Health Effects in Humans: A Review. *Environmental Science and Pollution Research*. 2014;21(20):11951–72.

141. Groth E, 3rd. Scientific Foundations of Fish Consumption Advice for Pregnant Women: Epidemiological Evidence, Benefit-risk Modeling, and an Integrated Approach. *Environ Res*. 2017;152:386–406.

142. Taylor CA-O, Emmett PM, Emond AM, Golding J. A Review of Guidance on Fish Consumption in Pregnancy: Is it Fit for Purpose? (1475–2727 (Electronic)).

143. EFSA. Consequences for the Consumer of the Use of Vitamin A in Animal Nutrition. *EFSA Journal*. 2009;7(2):873.

144. WHO Nutrition Unit. Safe Vitamin A Dosage During Pregnancy and Lactation: Recommendations and Report of a Consultation. World Health Organization; 1998.

145. Strobel M, Tinz J, Biesalski HK. The Importance of Beta-carotene as a Source of Vitamin A with Special Regard to Pregnant and Breastfeeding Women. *Eur J Nutr*. 2007;46(1):11–20.

146. EFSA. Consequences for the Consumer of the Use of Vitamin A in Animal Nutrition. *EFSA Journal*. 873.

147. Garcia-Larsen V, Ierodiakonou D, Jarrold K, Cunha S, Chivinge J, Robinson Z, et al. Diet During Pregnancy and Infancy and Risk of Allergic or Autoimmune Disease: A Systematic Review and Meta-analysis. *PLOS Medicine*. 2018;15(2):e1002507.

148. Philip AGS, Saigal S. When Should We Clamp the Umbilical Cord? *NeoReviews*. 2004;5(4):e142.

149. Burns E. More Than Clinical Waste? Placenta Rituals Among Australian Home-birthing Women. *J Perinat Educ*. 2014;23(1):41–9.

150. Young. In Search of Human Placentophagy. *Ecology of Food and Nutrition*. 467–84.

151. Ober WB. Notes on Placentophagy. *Bull N Y Acad Med*. 1979;55(6):591–9.

152. Yoshida K, Yamashita H, Ueda M, Tashiro N. Postnatal Depression in Japanese Mothers and the Reconsideration of 'Satogaeri Bunben'. *Pediatri Int*. 2001;43(2):189–93.

153. Dennis C-L, Fung K, Grigoriadis S, Robinson GE, Romans S, Ross L. Traditional Postpartum Practices and Rituals: A Qualitative Systematic Review. *Women's Health*. 2007;3(4):487–502.

154. Middleton P, Gomersall JC, Gould JF, Shepherd E, Olsen SF, Makrides M. Omega-3 Fatty Acid Addition During Pregnancy. *Cochrane Database Syst Rev*. 2018;11(11):CD003402–CD.

155. Bernabé BP, Tussing-Humphreys L, Rackers HS, Welke L, Mantha A, Kimmel MC. Improving Mental Health for the Mother-Infant Dyad by Nutrition and the Maternal Gut Microbiome. *Gastroenterol Clin North Am*. 2019;48(3):433–45.

156. Ibid.

157. Picciano MF. Nutrient Composition of Human Milk. *Pediatric Clinics of North America*. 2001;48(1):53–67.

158. Hassiotou F, Hepworth AR, Metzger P, Tat Lai C, Trengove N, Hartmann PE, et al. Maternal and Infant Infections Stimulate a Rapid Leukocyte Response in Breast Milk. *Clin Transl Immunology*. 2013;2(4):e3–e.

159. Innis SM. Human Milk: Maternal Dietary Lipids and Infant Development. *Proceedings of the Nutrition Society*. 2007;66(3):397–404.

160. Ibid.

161. Keikha M, Bahreynian M, Saleki M, Kelishadi R. Macro- and Micronutrients of Human Milk Composition: Are They Related to Maternal Diet? A Comprehensive Systematic Review. *Breastfeeding Medicine*. 2017;12(9):517–27.

162. Rodríguez JM, Fernández L, Verhasselt V. The Gut-Breast Axis: Programming Health for Life. *Nutrients*. 2021;13(2):606.

163. Bardanzellu F, Peroni DG, Fanos V. Human Breast Milk: Bioactive Components, from Stem Cells to Health Outcomes. *Current Nutrition Reports*. 2020;9(1):1–13.

164. Monteban M. Maternal Knowledge and Use of Galactagogues in Andean Communities of Cusco, Peru. *Ethnobiology Letters*. 2017;8(1):81–9.

165. The Academy of Breastfeeding Medicine Protocol Committee. ABM Clinical Protocol #9: Use of Galactogogues in Initiating or Augmenting the Rate of Maternal Milk Secretion (First Revision January 2011). Breastfeeding Medicine. 2011;6(1):41–9.

166. Rajani PS, Martin H, Groetch M, Järvinen KM. Presentation and Management of Food Allergy in Breastfed Infants and Risks of Maternal Elimination Diets. *The Journal of Allergy and Clinical Immunology: In Practice*. 2020;8(1):52–67.

167. McGee H. *McGee on Food and Cooking*. London: Hodder & Stoughton; 2004.

168. Damanik R. Torbangun (Coleus amboinicus Lour): A Bataknese Traditional Cuisine Perceived as Lactagogue by Bataknese Lactating Women in Simalungun, North Sumatera, Indonesia. *J Hum Lact*. 2009;25(1):64–72.

169. Jane MP. Food Yields and Nutrient Analyses of the Three Sisters: A Haudenosaunee Cropping System. *Ethnobiology Letters*. 2016;7(1).

170. Prentice J. *Full Moon Feast*. Vermont: Chelsea Green Publishing; 2006.

171. Miller KB, Hurst WJ, Payne MJ, Stuart DA, Apgar J, Sweigart DS, Ou B, et al. Impact of Alkalization on the Antioxidant and Flavanol Content of Commercial Cocoa Powders. *J Agric Food Chem*. 2008;56(18):8527–33.

172. Haggarty P. Fatty Acid Supply to the Human Fetus. *Annu Rev Nutr*. 2010;30:237–55.

173. Stark AH, Reifen R, Crawford MA. Past and Present Insights on Alpha-linolenic Acid and the Omega-3 Fatty Acid Family. *Critical Reviews in Food Science and Nutrition*. 2016;56(14):2261–7.

174. Ibid.

175. Crawford MA, Leigh Broadhurst C, Guest M, Nagar A, Wang Y, Ghebremeskel K, et al. A Quantum Theory for the Irreplaceable Role of Docosahexaenoic Acid in Neural Cell Signalling Throughout Evolution. *Prostaglandins, Leukotrienes and Essential Fatty Acids*. 2013;88(1):5–13.

176. Ibid.

177. Stark. Past and Present Insights on Alpha-linolenic Acid and the Omega-3 Fatty Acid Family. *Critical Reviews in Food Science and Nutrition*. 2261–7.

178. Bradbury J. Docosahexaenoic acid (DHA): An Ancient Nutrient for the Modern Human Brain. *Nutrients*. 2011;3(5):529–54.

179. Panth N, Gavarkovs A, Tamez M, Mattei J. The Influence of Diet on Fertility and the Implications for Public Health Nutrition in the United States. *Frontiers in Public Health*. 2018;6:211.

180. Mumford SL, Chavarro JE, Zhang C, Perkins NJ, Sjaarda LA, Pollack AZ, et al. Dietary Fat Intake and Reproductive Hormone Concentrations and Ovulation in Regularly Menstruating Women. *Am J Clin Nutr*. 2016;103(3):868–77.

181. Panth. The Influence of Diet on Fertility and the Implications for Public Health Nutrition in the United States. *Frontiers in Public Health*. 211.

182. Esmaeili V, Shahverdi AH, Moghadasian MH, Alizadeh AR. Dietary Fatty Acids Affect Semen Quality: A Review. *Andrology*. 2015;3(3):450–61.

183. Wathes DC, Abayasekara DRE, Aitken RJ. Polyunsaturated Fatty Acids in Male and Female Reproduction. *Biology of Reproduction*. 2007;77(2):190–201.

184. Daley CA, Abbott A, Doyle PS, Nader GA, Larson S. A Review of Fatty Acid Profiles and Antioxidant Content in Grass-fed and Grain-fed Beef. *Nutr J*. 2010;9:10–.

185. Rasmussen BF, Ennis MA, Dyer RA, Lim K, Elango R. Glycine, a Dispensable Amino Acid, is Conditionally Indispensable in Late Stages of Human Pregnancy. *The Journal of Nutrition*. 2021;151(2):361–9.

186. Hardy K, Brand-Miller J, Brown KD, Thomas MG, Copeland L. The Importance of Dietary Carbohydrate in Human Evolution. Q Rev Biol. 2015 Sep;90(3):251–68.

187. Ibid.

188. Zhong M, Kawaguchi R, Kassai M, Sun H. Retina, Retinol, Retinal and the Natural History of Vitamin A as a Light Sensor. *Nutrients*. 2012;4(12):2069–96.

189. Sokolovskaya OM, Shelton AN, Taga ME. Sharing Vitamins: Cobamides Unveil Microbial Interactions. *Science*. 2020;369(6499):eaba0165.

190. Ohta Y, Nishikimi M. Random Nucleotide Substitutions in Primate Non-functional Gene for l-gulono-gamma-lactone Oxidase, the Missing Enzyme in l-ascorbic acid Biosynthesis. *Biochimica et Biophysica Acta (BBA) — General Subjects*. 1999;1472(1):408–11.

191. Muscogiuri. Shedding New Light on Female Fertility. *Reviews in Endocrine and Metabolic Disorders*. 273–83.

192. Yuen AWC, Jablonski NG. Vitamin D: In the Evolution of Human Skin Colour. *Medical Hypotheses*. 2010;74(1):39–44.

193. Ibid.

194. Jarrett PΛ-O, Scragg R. Evolution, Prehistory and Vitamin D. *Int J Environ Res Public Health*. 2020;17(2):646.

195. Wolf G. The Discovery of the Antioxidant Function of Vitamin E: The Contribution of Henry A. Mattill. *The Journal of Nutrition*. 2005;135(3):363–6.

196. Olausson H, Goldberg GR, Ann Laskey M, Schoenmakers I, Jarjou LMA, Prentice A. Calcium Economy in Human Pregnancy and Lactation. *Nutrition Research Reviews*. 2012;25(1):40–67.

197. Movassagh EZ, Vatanparast H. Current Evidence on the Association of Dietary Patterns and Bone Health: A Scoping Review. *Advances in Nutrition*. 2017;8(1):1–16.

198. Eaton SB, Nelson DA. Calcium in Evolutionary Perspective. *Am J Clin Nutr*. 1991;54(1):281S– 7S.

199. Delshad H, Azizi F. Iodine Nutrition in Pregnant and Breastfeeding Women: Sufficiency, Deficiency, and Supplementation. *Hormones* (Athens). 2020;19(2):179–86.

200. Bath SC. The Effect of Iodine Deficiency During Pregnancy on Child Development. *Proceedings of the Nutrition Society*. 2019;78(2):150–60.

201. Yun AJ, Lee PY, Bazar KA, Daniel SM, Doux JD. The Incorporation of Iodine in Thyroid Hormone May Stem From its Role as a Prehistoric Signal of Ecologic Opportunity: An Evolutionary Perspective and Implications for Modern Diseases. *Medical Hypotheses*. 2005;65(4):804–10.

202. Kopp W. Nutrition, Evolution and Thyroid Hormone Levels — A Link to Iodine Deficiency Disorders? *Med Hypotheses*. 2004;62(6):871–5.

203. Keestra S, Vedrana T, Alvergne A. Reinterpreting Patterns of Variation in Human Thyroid Function: An Evolutionary Perspective. *Evolution, Medicine, and Public Health*. 2021;9(1):93– 112.

204. Smyth PPA, Burns R, Huang RJ, Hoffman T, Mullan K, Graham U, et al. Does Iodine Gas Released From Seaweed Contribute to Dietary Iodine Intake? *Environmental Geochemistry and Health*. 2011;33(4):389–97.

205. Duntas LA-O. Selenium and At-risk Pregnancy: Challenges and Controversies. *Thyroid Res*. 2020;12:16.

206. Qazi IH, Angel C, Yang H, Zoidis E, Pan B, Wu Z, et al. Role of Selenium and Selenoproteins in Male Reproductive Function: A Review of Past and Present Evidences. *Antioxidants* (Basel). 2019;8(8):268.

207. Salas-Huetos A, Rosique-Esteban N, Becerra-Tomás N, Vizmanos B, Bulló M, Salas- Salvadó J. The Effect of Nutrients and Dietary Supplements on Sperm Quality Parameters: A Systematic Review and Meta-Analysis of Randomized Clinical Trials. *Advances in Nutrition*. 2018;9(6):833–48.

208. Steiner AZ, Hansen KR, Barnhart KT, Cedars MI, Legro RS, Diamond MP, et al. The Effect of Antioxidants on Male Factor Infertility: The Males, Antioxidants, and Infertility (MOXI) Randomized Clinical Trial. *Fertil Steril*. 2020;113(3):552–560.e3.

209. Oldfield JE. *Selenium World Atlas*. Grimbergen, Belgium: Se-Tellurium Development Association (STDA). 1999.

210. Terrin G, Berni Canani R, Di Chiara M, Pietravalle A, Aleandri V, Conte F, et al. Zinc in Early Life: A Key Element in the Fetus and Preterm Neonate. *Nutrients*. 2015;7(12):10427–46.

211. Zlotkin SH, Cherian MG. Hepatic Metallothionein as a Source of Zinc and Cysteine During the First Year of Life. *Pediatr Res*. 1988;24(3):326–9.

212. Sandstead HH, Freeland-Graves JH. Dietary Phytate, Zinc and Hidden Zinc Deficiency. *Journal of Trace Elements in Medicine and Biology*. 2014;28(4):414–7.

213. Petroski W, Minich DA-O. Is There Such a Thing as 'Anti-Nutrients'? A Narrative Review of Perceived Problematic Plant Compounds. *Nutrients*. 2020;12(10):2929.

214. Muscogiuri. Shedding New Light on Female Fertility. *Reviews in Endocrine and Metabolic Disorders*. 273–83.

215. Chu J, Gallos I, Tobias A, Tan B, Eapen A, Coomarasamy A. Vitamin D and Assisted Reproductive Treatment Outcome: A Systematic Review and Meta-analysis. *Human Reproduction*. 2018;33(1):65–80.

216. Ozkan S, Jindal S, Greenseid K, Shu J, Zeitlian G, Hickman C, et al. Replete Vitamin D Stores Predict Reproductive Success Following In Vitro Fertilization. *Fertil Steril*. 2010;94(4):1314–19.

217. Panth. The Influence of Diet on Fertility and the Implications for Public Health Nutrition in the United States. *Frontiers in Public Health*. 211.

218. Heyden EL, Wimalawansa SJ. Vitamin D: Effects on Human Reproduction, Pregnancy, and Fetal Well-being. *The Journal of Steroid Biochemistry and Molecular Biology*. 2018;180:41–50.

219. Scientific Advisory Committee on Nutrition (SACN). *Vitamin D and Health*. Public Health England. 2016.

220. Australian Government Department of Health. *Clinical Practice Guidelines: Pregnancy Care* (Vitamin D). 2019.
221. National Health and Medical Research Council. *Iodine Supplementation for Pregnant and Breastfeeding Women*. 2010.
222. Innis. Human Milk. *Proceedings of the Nutrition Society*. 397–404.
223. Robson SL. Breast Milk, Diet, and Large Human Brains. *Current Anthropology*. 2004;45(3):419–25.
224. Davey GK, Spencer EA, Appleby PN, Allen NE, Knox KH, Key TJ. EPIC-Oxford: Lifestyle Characteristics and Nutrient Intakes in a Cohort of 33,883 Meat-eaters and 31,546 Non-meat-eaters in the UK. *Public Health Nutr*. 2003;6(3):259–69.
225. Bailey SW, Ayling JE. The Pharmacokinetic Advantage of 5-methyltetrahydrofolate for Minimization of the Risk for Birth Defects. *Sci Rep*. 2018;8(1):4096.
226. Panth. The Influence of Diet on Fertility and the Implications for Public Health Nutrition in the United States. *Frontiers in Public Health*. 211.
227. McNulty HA-O, Ward M, Hoey L, Hughes CF, Pentieva K. Addressing Optimal Folate and Related B-vitamin Status Through the Lifecycle: Health Impacts and Challenges. *Proc Nutr Soc*. 2019;78(3):449–462.
228. Scaglione. Folate, Folic Acid and 5-methyltetrahydrofolate are not the Same Thing. *Xenobiotica*. 480–8.
229. Bailey. The Pharmacokinetic Advantage of 5-methyltetrahydrofolate for Minimization of the Risk for Birth Defects. *Sci Rep*. 4096.
230. Rima O, Wolfgang H, Klaus P. Is 5-methyltetrahydrofolate an Alternative to Folic Acid for the Prevention of Neural Tube Defects? *Journal of Perinatal Medicine*. 2013;41(5):469–83.
231. Servy EJ, Jacquesson-Fournols L, Cohen M, Menezo YJR. MTHFR Isoform Carriers. 5-MTHF (5-methyl tetrahydrofolate) vs Folic Acid: A Key to Pregnancy Outcome: A Case Series. *J Assist Reprod Genet*. 2018;35(8):1431–5.
232. Scaglione. Folate, Folic Acid and 5-methyltetrahydrofolate are not the Same Thing. *Xenobiotica*. 480–8.
233. Ferrazzi E, Tiso G, Di Martino D. Folic Acid Versus 5-methyltetrahydrofolate Supplementation in Pregnancy. *European Journal of Obstetrics & Gynecology and Reproductive Biology*. 2020.
234. O'Donnell A, McParlin C, Robson SC, Beyer F, Moloney E, Bryant A, et al. Treatments for Hyperemesis Gravidarum and Nausea and Vomiting in Pregnancy: A Systematic Review and Economic Assessment. *Health Technol Assess*. 2016;20(74).
235. Bailey. The Pharmacokinetic Advantage of 5-methyltetrahydrofolate for Minimization of the Risk for Birth Defects. *Sci Rep*. 4096.
236. Rodriguez-Diaz E, Pearce EN. Iodine Status and Supplementation Before, During, and After Pregnancy. *Best Pract Res Clin Endocrinol Metab*. 2020;34(4):101430.
237. Delshad. Iodine Nutrition in Pregnant and Breastfeeding Women. *Hormones*. 179–86.
238. Rodriguez-Diaz. Iodine Status and Supplementation Before, During, and After Pregnancy. *Best Pract Res Clin Endocrinol Metab*. 101430.
239. Zimmermann MB. Iodine Supplements for Mildly Iodine-deficient Pregnant Women: Are They Worthwhile? *Am J Clin Nutr*. 2020;112(2):247–8.
240. Bath. The Effect of Iodine Deficiency During Pregnancy on Child Development. *Proceedings of the Nutrition Society*. 150–60.
241. Dineva M, Fishpool H, Rayman MP, Mendis J, Bath SC. Systematic Review and Meta-analysis of the Effects of Iodine Supplementation on Thyroid Function and Child Neurodevelopment in Mildly-to-moderately Iodine-deficient Pregnant Women. *Am J Clin Nutr*. 2020;112(2):389–412.
242. Fisher AL, Nemeth E. Iron Homeostasis During Pregnancy. *Am J Clin Nutr*. 2017;106(Suppl 6):1567S–74S.
243. Miller. The Reproductive Ecology of Iron in Women. *Am J Phys Anthropol*. S172–96.
244. Ibid.
245. Weinberg ED. Can Iron be Teratogenic? *Biometals*. 2010;23(2):181–4.
246. Domellöf M. Iron Requirements, Absorption and Metabolism in Infancy and Childhood. *Current Opinion in Clinical Nutrition & Metabolic Care*. 2007;10(3).
247. Miller. The Reproductive Ecology of Iron in Women. *Am J Phys Anthropol*. S172–96.

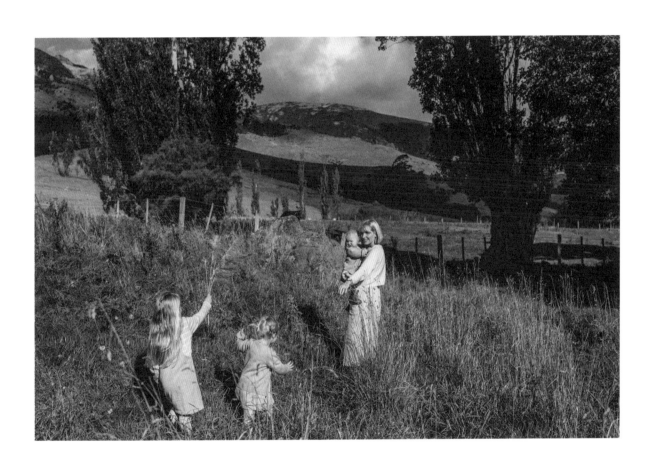

INDEX

RECIPES

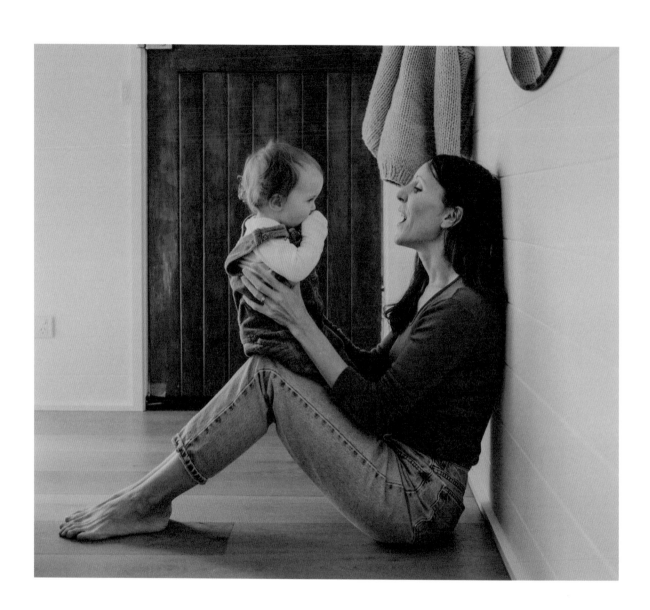

Acknowledgments

I wrote this book during the beginnings of the tumultuous time of upheaval stirred by the wake of the Covid-19 pandemic. A time when life as we knew it began to shift — rapidly and irreversibly. Yet, amidst the liminal times of uncertainty and chaos came a growing awareness that our lifeways are not fenced in but open. And that the wilds beyond the imaginary fences that we have mentally constructed for ourselves are awash with possibilities. Life, as motherhood also teaches us, can be otherwise.

I will be forever indebted to my children, who remind me every day of why it is so important to see beyond the fences that hold us in our ways. My journey on this path of unravelling and reweaving began with them. Rob — you made this possible, and together with my friends and family, provide me with enduring love and support as we walk out into the wilds. Thank you.

Thanks to Vicki for continuing this journey with me and connecting me with the wonderful team at Bateman — Sam, Louise and Paul, whose patience and flexibility meant that the words finally made it out beyond *my* fences. Thanks to Megan for your beautiful and considered design and to Rosanna for complimenting this with your heartfelt art — the food activism work you do through your craft is an inspiration. To Jacinta for your photography and styling and ability to laugh at the futility of planning anything in the chaos of the pandemic. Thanks to Phil, Anne and Eman for helping with cooking, cleaning and styling on the shoots. To Olivia and Danielle for your photography that beautifully captures motherhood's transitionary essence in a single moment — and to all the mothers that granted us the opportunity to see these precious glimpses.

If we are to rematriate our foodways, it will be a collective effort. Contrary to what is often thought, matriarchy does not mean the dominance of women over men but an entirely different way of life. A life not even based on hierarchies and domination, but one that is woven with an appreciation for our interdependence. So, I want to thank you for reading this book — because without you it wouldn't exist. I hope that your journey into the wilds of motherhood is joyful and illuminating, but most of all rooted in connection.

About the Author

Before the birth of her first child, Vanessa A. Clarkson attained a first-class honours degree in dietetics and a masters degree with distinction in food policy. She worked with governments, public agencies, non-profit organisations, academic institutions and food businesses and felt sure of what needed to be done to instil a regenerative human presence on Earth. More than ten years ago, Vanessa commenced her journey from these familiar grounds into the uncertain and wild terrains of motherhood. Over the next decade of unravelling and reweaving, Vanessa has embarked on a journey of reflection on her foodways, questioning humanity's response to the crises that entangle civilisation. *Motherfood* is part of Vanessa's response to that questioning. Since writing *Motherfood*, her second book, Vanessa has begun her PhD on food system transitions at the University of Melbourne. Her first book, *Real Food for Babies and Toddlers*, won the *Smallish Parenting* magazine award for Best Family Cookbook. Vanessa lives with her husband and three boys on unceded Boon Wurrung Country in Victoria, Australia.

Text © Vanesssa A. Clarkson, 2022
The moral rights of the author have been asserted.
Typographical design © David Bateman Ltd, 2022

Published in 2022 by David Bateman Ltd,
Unit 2/5 Workspace Drive, Hobsonville,
Auckland 0618, New Zealand
www.batemanbooks.co.nz
ISBN: 978-1-77689-017-0

A catalogue record for this book is available from the National Library of New Zealand.

Book design: Megan van Staden
Woodcut illustrations: Rosanna Morris
Food photography: Jacinta Moore
Photography by Olivia van Leeuwen: 16–17, 28–29, 87, 103, 105–107, 130–131, 133, 134, 136–137, 139, 141, 143, 274–275, 291, 294–295, 300.
Photography by Danielle Dobson: 7, 62–63, 75, 94, 307.
Unsplash: 14, 23, 43
Index by Anna Corballis Fry

Printed in China by Everbest Printing Co. Ltd

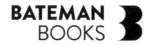

BATEMAN BOOKS